THE

Patient's Guide to

OUTSTANDING
BREAST CANCER
CARE

THE
Patient's Guide to

OUTSTANDING
BREAST CANCER
CARE

EDITED BY
GREGORY SENOFSKY, M.D., F.A.C.S., F.S.S.O.,
WITH LAUREN HARTMAN

A Perigee Book

Every effort has been made to ensure that the information contained in this book is complete and accurate. However, neither the publisher nor the author is engaged in rendering professional advice or services to the individual reader. The ideas, procedures, and suggestions contained in this book are not intended as a substitute for consulting with your physician. All matters regarding your health require medical supervision. Neither the author nor the publisher shall be liable or responsible for any loss or damage allegedly arising from any information or suggestion in this book.

A Perigee Book
Published by The Berkley Publishing Group
A division of Penguin Putnam Inc.
375 Hudson Street
New York, New York 10014

First edition: September 2002

Visit our website at www.penguinputnam.com

Library of Congress Cataloging-in-Publication Data

Senofsky, Greg.
    The patient's guide to outstanding breast cancer care / Gregory Senofsky, with Lauren Hartman.
        p.   cm.
    Includes bibliographical references and index.
    ISBN 0-399-52811-3
    1. Breast—Cancer—Popular works. I. Title: Outstanding breast cancer care. II. Hartman, Lauren. III. Title.

    RC280.B8 S46 2002
    616.99'449—dc21

                                                                    2002025240

Printed in the United States of America

10   9   8   7   6   5   4   3   2   1

I would like to dedicate this book to
Tanya, Nicholas, Shirley, Berl, Sloan, and Brandi.

Contents

ABOUT THE AUTHORS

Gregory Senofsky, M.D., F.A.C.S., F.S.S.O., is the Founder and Surgical Director of The Breast Institute, which has three locations in the greater Los Angeles area (Valencia, Tarzana, and Lancaster). He has authored numerous medical publications on breast cancer and lectured extensively, and is an active breast cancer surgeon, Assistant Clinical Professor of Surgery at UCLA School of Medicine, Affiliate Breast Surgeon to Women's Cancer Centers, and the Medical Director of The Breast Cancer Resource Center, a not-for-profit foundation.

Lauren Hartman is the author of *Solutions: The Woman's Crisis Handbook.*

CONTRIBUTORS

John Barstis, M.D., is Associate Clinical Professor of Medicine at UCLA Center for Health Sciences in Los Angeles and Medical Director of UCLA Cancer Centers at Santa Clarita and Antelope Valley in California. Dr. Barstis has published extensively in clinical journals and textbooks.

Alexander C. Black, M.D., is Associate Clinical Professor, UCLA School of Medicine, Associate Director of UCLA/SCV Cancer Centers in California, and American Board of Internal Medicine (ABIM) certified in internal medicine, medical oncology, and hematology. Dr. Black has over 20 publications in basic science and clinical journals and textbooks.

Maurice Cohen, M.D., F.A.C.S., F.A.C.O.G., F.A.C.E., has spent much of his four-decade professional life dedicated to women's health issues and is considered a pioneer in the area of women's health at midlife. He serves as Consultant for the Women's Health Program at ProHealth Care Associates in Lake Success, New York, and is an attending physician with the North Shore-LIJ Health System at Long Island Jewish Medical Center in New Hyde Park, New York.

William Colburn, M.D., is Chief Pathologist and Codirector of Laboratories at the Encino-Tarzana Medical Center in Tarzana, California. He is a nationally known breast pathologist with over 60 publication contributions and abstracts to his credit.

William C. Dooley, M.D., F.A.C.S., is a G. Rainey Williams Professor of Surgical Oncology and the Director of the University of Okalahoma Breast Institute. Dr. Dooley is a leader in patient satisfaction–driven care, patient empowerment, and the new ductal approach to the screening and treatment of breast cancer.

Seth P. Harlow, M.D., is a principal investigator for the University of Vermont, National Surgical Adjuvant Breast and Bowel Project, Surgical Training Chair for NSABP B32 protocol, and a contributor to numerous publications, particularly in the area of sentinel node biopsy.

Judith Harris, M.A., M.F.T., is Director of Attitudinal Healing Associates in Chatsworth, California. Trained as a teacher and psychotherapist, Ms. Harris blends humor, psychology, and cultural observations in a unique and powerful way to help us understand how we become who we are. She has facilitated groups for AIDS Project L.A., and the American Cancer Society, and currently leads caregiver, bereavement, and stress groups.

J. Arthur Jensen, M.D., is Assistant Clinical Professor of Plastic Surgery at UCLA School of Medicine and a plastic surgeon in private practice in Santa Monica, California. Dr. Jensen has authored numerous articles on breast reconstruction and is an expert in TRAM flap reconstruction.

Daniel Kirsch, M.D., is Staff Radiologist and Director of Breast Imaging, Valencia Imaging Medical Group and Assistant Professor of Radiology, Breast Imaging Specialist, Clinical Faculty of UCLA Medical Center.

Claudia Z. Lee, M.B.A., is President of C. Z. Lee & Associates and has been an administrator of two comprehensive breast centers. Ms. Lee has consulted with approximately one hundred institutions and physician groups in their efforts to develop comprehensive breast programs.

Bernard S. Lewinsky, M.D., F.A.C.R., is a radiation oncologist and Director and President of Western Tumor Medical Group in Sherman Oaks, California, which treats all types of cancer, including breast cancer. Dr. Lewinsky is Clinical Assistant Professor in Radiation Oncology at UCLA. His abstracts and publication credits number in the sixties, and he has written three textbook chapters on breast cancer.

Michelle B. Riba, M.D., M.S., is the Director of the Psycho-Oncology Program at the University of Michigan Comprehensive Cancer Center, Associate Chair for Education and Academic Affairs, Clinical Associate Professor of Psychiatry, Department of Psychiatry at the University of Michigan, and Consulting Psychiatrist to the University of Michigan Multidisciplinary Breast Cancer Center and Melanoma Clinic.

Steven M. Rosman, Ph.D., L.A.c., M.S., D.A.P.A., is Director, Division of Complementary Medicine at ProHealth Care Associates in Lake Success, New York, where he practices acupuncture, Oriental medicine, Eastern and Western nutrition, herbal and botanical medicine, quigong, and lifestyle counseling. He is an internationally known speaker, motivator, and the author of ten books including *Jewish Healing Wisdom* and *Jewish Parenting Wisdom.*

Howard Singer, M.D., is Medical Director of Anesthesia and Pain Management at Henry Mayo Newhall Memorial Hospital in Valencia, California, and is board certified by the American Board of Anesthesiology.

Ellen Tobin, M.ed., is President of Cancer Care Strategies and a professional focus group moderator. She has facilitated more than twenty-five hundred cancer-related focus groups and has conducted nearly a thousand focus groups with breast cancer patients. She is a cancer survivor.

FOREWORD

A diagnosis of breast cancer often creates confusion, uncertainty, and a feeling of loss of control. One way that a woman can regain control of her life is to participate in making decisions about her treatment. To do this, she needs acccurate information about treatment options and possible outcomes.

This comprehensive, state-of-the-art book provides the information you need to work with your doctor to identify treatment goals and weigh the benefits, risks, and possible consequences of various treatments. Because each patient is unique, and because medical care for breast disease is constantly evolving, building a plan for treatment is a complex process. The authors, who are breast cancer specialists, serve as your personal advocates in sorting through medical advice. Where appropriate, controversial approaches are addressed and opposing types of treatment are discussed. Throughout the book, you will find quotes from former breast cancer patients. The women describe in their own words their experiences and feelings during and after treatment.

By becoming an active partner in your health care team, the fear of breast cancer is replaced with the knowledge that you are still in charge of your body and the important priorities in your life.

—S. Eva Singletary, M.D., F.A.C.S.
   Professor of Surgery,
   Department of Surgical Oncology,
   Chief Section of Breast Cancer 1990–2000,
   The University of Texas, MD Anderson Cancer Center
   and
   Chair, American Joint Commission on Cancer (AJCC) Breast Task
   Force

ACKNOWLEDGMENTS

I would like to thank the following doctors for helping to shape my thinking and operative techniques in the field of breast cancer surgery:

Alfred Ketchum, M.D.

Melvin J. Silverstein, M.D.

Richard Davies, M.D.

Harold Wanebo, M.D.

J. Arthur Jensen, M.D.

Parvis Gamagami, M.D.

INTRODUCTION

Gregory Senofsky, M.D., F.A.C.S, F.S.S.O.

When discussing the Great Depression, Franklin Delano Roosevelt once said, "The only thing we have to fear is fear itself." I strongly urge any woman or man (about 1 out of 100 cases of breast cancer occur in men) who thinks they may have a small change in their breast or under their arm to see a physician well-versed in diagnosing breast cancer immediately. Do not let the fear of possible breast cancer keep you from seeking appropriate medical attention or, for that matter, from having your yearly mammograms (beginning at age 40) and physical examinations. A breast cancer diagnosis is an urgent, but not emergent, situation. You have time to seek expert professional care. You should begin seeking medical attention immediately after you identify a change in your breast. Biopsy, if indicated, should be done within two to three weeks following consultation with your physician.

The information you are about to read in this book could make the process of diagnosis and treatment significantly better for you. I created and edited this book because breast cancer treatment has evolved into an area of true specialization, and the standards of excellence for breast cancer diagnosis and treatment can differ, depending on whether your doctor truly specializes in this field of medicine. I handpicked noted experts in the field to acquaint you with the highest standards of current practice in breast cancer care and to help you understand what your best options may be, knowing that the best choice for care can vary for each woman. The medical specialists who contributed to this book are university-affiliated doctors who are on the front lines of breast cancer treatment and who are widely published in their fields. Yet, you will find the chapters easy to read and the concepts simple to grasp, as each contributor is committed to helping patients with breast cancer attain the best care possible.

This book covers the entire diagnosis and treatment process to help you determine what to do if you feel a lump or change in your breast or if you are told that you have an abnormal mammogram. You'll learn about newer techniques that allow surgeons to remove a good-sized abnormality in the breast without significantly changing its appearance or to remove a breast cancer along with a significant rim of healthy breast tissue around it (called the *margin of clearance*) to greatly reduce the chance that the cancer will come back in the breast and, at the same time, leave the breast looking similar, and sometimes even better, than before surgery. In the case of mastectomy, you will learn about options for skin sparing, about the possibility of immediate breast reconstruction after mastectomy, and about the advantages of having the plastic surgeon and breast surgeon work together to plan and perform surgery as a team. You will find information about chemotherapy, including new drugs that can significantly reduce the side effects of chemotherapy as well as treatments to reduce any pain that you experience. You'll read about hormone therapy, the stages of breast cancer, and managing recurrent breast cancer. Sentinel node biopsy, a new, less-intrusive surgery performed to determine whether cancer has spread to the lymph nodes, will also be covered. We'll talk about what's new in radiotherapy treatment and about the critical role the pathologist plays in your treatment. Because many people are uncertain about anesthesia, we've also included a chapter to help you understand the various options for anesthesia, depending on the type of surgery you will have and what your preferences are.

The relationship between estrogen and breast cancer, and questions about hormone therapy are addressed, and we will take an in-depth look at new diet and lifestyle strategies for optimum breast health. Finally, we will talk about your emotions and relationships after a breast cancer diagnosis, about dealing with a life-threatening disease, and the information you need to choose and evaluate your doctors or an organized breast program. You will also hear directly from women who have had breast cancer and who have been gracious enough to provide other women with their insights about dealing with medical decisions, changes in relationships, and other emotional and psychological issues related to the battle against a life-threatening illness.

The contributors to this book believe that the best approach to breast cancer care and treatment is the team approach. When the surgical oncologist, medical oncologist, pathologist, radiation oncologist, radiologist, and anesthesiologist all work together with other important team members, patients with breast cancer can receive the highest level of breast cancer care and treatment available. You *can* get through this. But you will need courage and information. We'll do our best to provide you with both.

CHAPTER ONE

You've Just Discovered
a Breast Lump

By Gregory Senofsky, M.D., F.A.C.S., F.S.S.O.

What I felt was hard and pea shaped. That evening I willed my hand to touch the spot and have the lump be gone. It didn't work. I felt a chill go through me that never went away. • Diane

I went in for my regular check up with my OB-GYN and she said, "Everything is fine. The lump in your breast hasn't grown." I said, "Excuse me?" I found out I had a lump that my OB-GYN and surgeon said was probably benign. Although the surgeon said we usually just leave it alone, I stressed that I wanted it out. Things were changing at my company, and I thought I might not have insurance later on. • Janice

All I could think about was how stupid I felt. The mass I had was so big. How could I have not felt it before? How long had it been since I really checked? Why did it take me so long to find it? I felt incredibly alone and empty. • Cynthia

If you have noticed a lump or a small change in your breast or under your arm, you may be feeling anxious, overwhelmed, and frightened. It's normal to worry and to be scared, because a breast abnormality is a potentially serious situation, although most breast lumps discovered by women turn out to be benign. However, it's important to have any lump evaluated by a specialist who has the ability to fully assess breast lumps in order to distinguish between those that are more of a concern and those that are likely to be benign. This may be your gynecologist or a breast surgeon. (See page 7.)

All Breast Lumps Are Not Alike

Many women have lumpy/gravelly or fibrocystic breasts, which may be painful or tender, especially before the menstrual period. You are more likely to develop fibrocystic breasts in late or early womanhood. (Your gynecologist will recognize this condition and apprise you of it, if you have it.) In the hands of an experienced examiner, most fibrocystic lumps do not signal red flags; however, they can pose diagnostic challenges. Dense fibrocystic breasts appear white on a mammogram, as will a breast cancer, thus there is the dangerous possibility that a fibrocystic breast condition will hide a breast cancer on a mammogram. Ultrasound may also be less reliable for some fibrocystic conditions. If you have fibrocystic breasts, it's crucial that you become familiar with their internal contours by monthly breast self-exams so that you can identify any changes.

Painful or tender fibrocystic breasts can improve if you stop consuming chocolate and beverages containing caffeine. Quitting caffeine can be tough, but there are many health benefits, one of which can be reducing the lumpiness and pain in your breasts. I also find that vitamin E and oil of evening primrose can lessen lumpiness. I prescribe 400 IU of vitamin E twice a day and 500 milligrams of oil of evening primrose twice a day. Both are available in capsule form over the counter. It's also important to know that oral estrogens, such as birth control pills or hormone replacement therapy, can intensify fibrocystic breast lumps in some cases.

If you have fibrocystic breasts, I suggest that you take a look at Chapter 5, "Are You at Risk for Late Diagnosis?," for some additional information. I would advise you to be wary of a physician who too easily dismisses your concerns about a breast lump.

It's also possible that an inexperienced examiner will overlook a cancer in severely fibrocystic breasts, attributing it to part of a fibrocystic condition. If there is any question that you might in fact have a tumor, an experienced physician will order tests beyond a mammogram and ultrasound, such as a fine needle aspiration or core needle biopsy. At the very minimum, I will do a fine needle aspiration for a woman with fibrocystic breasts who comes to see me with a new lump in her breast. Fine needle aspiration is a type of biopsy in which your physician uses a very thin needle to withdraw cells from the lump for analysis. The needle is so thin it can't be used to draw blood. The procedure is usually done in the office without local anesthetic (because it interferes with the processing of the cells). It

WHAT TO LOOK FOR IN A BREAST SURGEON

Make sure that breast cancer surgery comprises at least 75 percent of your surgeon's practice.

Why a Breast Surgeon?

Breast surgeons have additional training beyond general surgery that includes a fellowship in surgical oncology or a one-year fellowship in breast surgery. Surgical oncology fellowships typically confer significant added exposure to breast cancer surgery in all of its detail. There is currently no specific board certification in breast surgery. Look for a surgeon who is at least board certified in general surgery.

For more information on choosing physicians, see chapter 19, "How to Get the Best Care and Treatment."

doesn't typically hurt, but you may feel a pinch when the needle is inserted and mild discomfort. Alternatives to fine needle aspiration include core needle biopsy, which we'll discuss below, or cosmetic removal of the lump, which will then be sent to the pathology lab for analysis.

Young women often have lumps that are very round and move easily within the breast upon examination. These lumps, called *fibroadenomas*, are more typical in young women in their teens through their thirties, although women in their forties and fifties can have them too. Here again, there is a danger that a doctor may dismiss a small, round breast cancer in a young woman as a fibroadenoma. If they are small and obvious as fibroadenomas, these lumps may be observed, but if there is any question, fine needle aspiration will reveal the benign microscopic nature of the cells in the lump. Fibroadenomas can grow, especially during periods of increased circulating estrogen in the body—for example, due to pregnancy or taking hormones—and they can become uncomfortable, so patients often request that mid- and large-sized fibroadenomas be removed through small cosmetic surgical incisions.

If You Find a New Lump in Your Breast

If you notice a new lump, see your primary care physician and an experienced breast surgeon for an evaluation. Going to a breast surgeon doesn't mean that you have, or are likely to have, breast cancer. A breast surgeon is simply the medical professional most likely to diagnose and treat your lump accurately. Your breast surgeon should devote at least 75 percent of his or her practice to breast surgery. In Chapter 19, "How to Find the Best Care and Treatment," you will locate more information on how to find and choose a breast surgeon.

| HMO SURVIVAL TIP

Make sure your biopsy and biopsy results are not being delayed by paperwork or a systems error. Your biopsy should be performed within two to three weeks of your decision to have it done. Your results should be in two to three days from the time you had your biopsy done.

Early detection is the key to survival, and I know I only have to look into the eyes of my five grandchildren to know I want to be around for a long time. I think I finally get it. Life isn't supposed to be easy or fair. Life is conquering the challenges that come along and learning the lessons. Life is living and then finding some way of giving back. • Dianne

Diagnosing a Breast Lump

Most breast lumps are not cancerous, but a breast cancer that is found early is more likely to be successfully treated than a cancer found later. That's why it is vital that you do not neglect a new lump. Adequate testing by a specialist must be done for a proper diagnosis. On your first visit, your breast surgeon should ask your age, when you first noticed the lump, if it is growing, and whether or not it is painful. A word of caution here: Try to be objective about the time at which you first noticed the lump. Fear can trick us into providing explanations for difficult facts, such as thinking that a lump is the result of trauma to the breast or has been present for a long time. Be honest with yourself. Is this a new lump? You and your physician will need to know. Patients must be truthful with their doctors. If a physician is told that the lump has been there for several years, he or she may be less inclined to recommend biopsy. Your breast surgeon will also ask you whether the lump changes with your menstrual cycle, if you are menstruating, and whether you notice any new nipple discharge. He or she should ask about your family history and your history of prior breast surgeries. You should have a full examination of both breasts, the area under your armpits (known as the axillae), and the area around your collarbone and neck. Your nipple must be examined for possible brown or bloody discharge or scaling of the skin, and the skin of your breasts should be examined for discoloration or changes in normal contour.

Generally, the first step in diagnosis is to determine whether the lump is solid or cystic (fluid-filled). There are two ways to do this: through ultrasound, a noninvasive method that uses sound waves to obtain images for diagnostic purposes, and fine needle aspiration.

Fine needle aspiration can be used to determine whether the lump is solid or cystic, depending on how obvious the lump is and how fibrocystic your breasts are. Ultrasound can be used as a diagnostic tool when the lump can't be easily distinguished or when it does not yield fluid, and a radiologist (a doctor who is trained to diagnose disease using imaging studies) can perform fine needle aspiration with ultrasound guidance, when necessary. (See Chapter 2, "You've Just Been Told That You Have an Abnormal Mammogram.") Most cysts are simple round cysts with smooth walls and liquid inside. These simple cysts can be left alone or drained with a needle, depending on your wishes. Cysts that cause discomfort or bulge can be easily aspirated.

The vast majority of cysts are benign. If the cyst yields clear fluid and completely dissolves on aspiration, you won't need further testing, but the cyst should be checked for redevelopment later on. If the cyst does not completely resolve, the remaining lump should be cosmetically removed and the fluid sent for cell analysis. Fluid from the cyst that is bloody or cloudy should be sent for analysis as, very rarely, this can be an indication of malignancy. If a cyst recurs two or three times after aspiration, it can be removed if bothersome through a tiny cosmetic incision that will not damage the appearance of the breast, if

> **BEFORE HAVING A CYST REMOVED, ASK YOUR SURGEON:**
>
> • What is the indication for surgery?
>
> • How long will my incision be?
>
> • How will my breast look after surgery?
>
> • Will my incision go in the direction of the natural skin lines of my breast? These are the lines of least tension, which will yield the thinnest and least noticeable scar.

done correctly. A surgeon should never use a large incision to remove a cyst. Occasionally, a cyst will be considered complex because it has a growth on the inner wall or solid material inside. The majority of complex cysts are benign; yet some types are of greater concern. Complex cysts that appear to be benign can be aspirated. They can also be cosmetically removed to prove conclusively that they are benign. If, by ultrasound, the complex cyst looks suspicious, I would not recommend aspiration, because if the cyst is cancerous, the cells can spread into the breast, and the remaining cancer can be difficult to identify radiographically after aspiration. Suspicious complex cysts should be surgically removed.

If you are over 35 and you have a solid lump in your breast, you should have a mammogram and, in general, an ultrasound. Once we know that the lump is solid, a decision must be made to further identify the nature of the lump. The easiest way to do this is through fine needle aspiration. I use this technique routinely on the vast majority of solid breast masses unless the mass is extremely deep and can't be found reliably by the tip of the needle in the office setting. In these cases, there is the option of doing ultrasound-guided or stereotactic core needle biopsy, which incorporates ultrasound or mammography, and which Dr. Kirsch will explain in the following chapter. Before we do an ultrasound or stereotactic core needle biopsy, we must be sure that it is safe to do the procedure. If the mass is extremely close to the chest wall, there is a danger that the needle could enter your chest.

If a fine needle aspiration of a solid lump is not suspicious for cancer, and the mammogram and ultrasound are not suspicious, you and your breast surgeon must decide whether or not to observe the lump, perform a core needle biopsy on the lump, or cosmetically remove the lump. Core needle biopsy is similar to fine needle biopsy, except that a significantly larger needle is used to obtain a sliver of tissue from the lump for analysis. (In Chapter 2, "You've Just Been Told That You Have an Abnormal Mammogram," you will read about core needle biopsies done by radiologists. In these circumstances, bigger needles are used and more cores are taken.) Core needle biopsy is done with a local anesthetic and can leave a small blemish on the breast. If multiple core needle biopsies are needed, I usually do them in an outpatient operating room with intravenous sedation. Core needle biopsy done by hand is different from image-guided core needle biopsy, which we discuss in the next chapter. No incision in the breast is necessary before a core needle biopsy done by hand.

There is a possibility of obtaining a false negative with a fine needle aspiration, and thus a core needle biopsy or cosmetic surgical excision can be used to verify or disprove the fine needle aspiration when the cytology (the microscopic appearance of the cells) result doesn't fit the appearance of the lesion. I use core needle biopsy as a preoperative tool to determine whether a breast lump is benign or malignant before removing it. Core needle biopsy is also helpful for ruling out cancer in large, hard thickenings likely to be fibrocystic changes.

Some women wish to bypass needle biopsies to go directly to surgical removal of a lump. This is certainly an option, although needle biopsies can provide valuable information to your surgeon. Once we have a diagnosis, we have the information we need to better plan the surgery, including how much tissue to remove along with the lump. If the lump is malignant, we can also plan a surgery called *sentinel node biopsy* to determine whether the cancer has spread to the lymph nodes. We can do that surgery first, then remove the lump with a margin or rim of normal tissue attached to it, making the entire procedure easier and quicker. (For more information about sentinel node biopsy, see Chapter 8, "Removing Lymph Nodes.")

Sometimes a woman will want to do a core needle biopsy, wait to see if the results are negative for cancer, and do no further surgery. This is reasonable *if* the pathology is completely benign, not premalignant, and there is no question that the core needle actually biopsied the lump. There is always a tiny possibility that the core needle will miss lump. The breast surgeon must make sure that the pathology analysis correlates to the way it appears on the mammogram or ultrasound to make sure that the lump was hit with the biopsy needle. It's also very

IF YOUR FINE NEEDLE BIOPSY IS SUSPICIOUS FOR CANCER

Fine needle aspirations are very accurate when positive for cancer and less so when negative. If you have had a fine needle aspiration that is suspicious for cancer, there is a high likelihood that you do have cancer, although you have the option of doing a core needle biopsy to further document and verify that fact.

I had a fine needle biopsy, and I knew that the results wouldn't be back until the following week. That was a very difficult week. But deep down in my heart, I think I knew. I think I knew that that year would be my year to fight. · Linda R.

I will talk to my patients about their surgical options for dealing with lumps up to one to one-and-a-half inches in diameter. These include core needle biopsy, excisional biopsy, wide excisional biopsy, or lumpectomy and possibly sentinel node mapping. These procedures are invasive, but can be performed on an outpatient basis. Women should be aware that breast surgery for breast cancer often requires radiation therapy treatment. I mention mastectomy as a possible option in the future should the need arise. Lumps larger than one to one-and-a-half inches in diameter usually require definitive needle biopsy prior to surgical treatment.

Some surgeons may proceed to core needle biopsy and watch the lump, if the core needle biopsy is negative. I find that after an abnormal fine needle aspiration, most women want the lump removed and most surgeons would agree with that.

important to correlate the pathologic results to the way the lump feels to the surgeon. Occasionally, this can be difficult because a small breast cancer can be surrounded by fibrocystic changes, and the diagnosis of fibrocystic changes can be considered a plausible pathologic finding. However, the lump can be a small breast cancer, the needle can miss it, and the result of fibrocystic changes can be accepted when the truth is that the cancer was not adequately biopsied. But again, this is an unusual situation.

In my practice, I find that most women with solid lumps want them cosmetically removed. Although most lumps are benign, the psychological stress and anxiety experienced with a palpable breast lump can be significant. Removal of a lump is certainly the safest and most psychologically calming option, because the lump is gone and its nature is thoroughly determined. In rare cases, a lump will turn out to be malignant despite an unsuspicious fine needle aspiration, mammogram, and ultrasound.

The Two Most Frequent Questions

The two questions my patients ask most frequently are "What will you do if the lump is malignant?" and "What will my breast look like after you take the lump out?" Removal of a small, clearly benign lump is done as an excisional biopsy. This is an outpatient operation performed while you are under deep sedation or general anesthesia. I typically remove the lump with a tiny rim or capsule of normal tissue. Unless extremely large, the removal of a benign lump should not significantly affect the breast, if done properly. The smallest possible incision in the natural skin lines should be used and the lump should be removed in its entirety.

You should have a very thin cosmetic scar, as small as possible in the natural skin lines, and no dimpling or puckering. It is very important that your surgeon examine you while you are awake preoperatively so that you can both find the lump together and put a mark on the skin with a marking pen exactly where the incision will be made. Surgeons must be cautious about how much local anesthetic they inject around the lump prior to its removal. Local anesthetic puffs the tissue out around the lump and can make it difficult to find the lump during surgery.

If during surgery it's discovered that the lump is a fibrocystic thickening rather than a discrete mass, mature surgical judgment should be used to determine how much of the thickening to take or remove based on prior discussions with

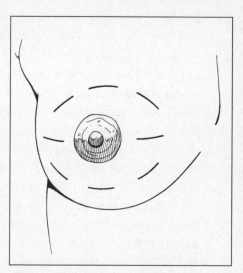

Figure 1. Orientation for local excision incisions.

you, the patient. Some women want their fibrocystic lumps removed, as some fibrocystic thickenings can be very pronounced. Again, it's obviously best not to change the shape of the breast during this procedure. Fibrocystic pain is generally treated best by nonsurgical approaches.

> *Most surgeons don't like to remove benign lumps, because they're afraid they'll leave a scar. All I have is about a one- to two-centimeter scar that looks like a scratch. I have no lumps now. I know that in time the scratch will probably disappear.* • Janice

> *I have a very slight scar. It looks completely natural. I am thrilled with the cosmetic outcome of my breast cancer surgery.* • Anne

If you have a large lump and small- to medium-sized breasts, it is more difficult to take out the lump without causing some deformity to the breast. A newer surgical technique (one that is not new to plastic surgeons) called *flap advancement* can prevent or reduce any potential indentation of the breast after the lump is removed, whether it is benign or malignant. This technique involves gently separating the back edges of the breast at the edges of the lumpectomy from the surface of the chest muscles in order to release the back edges and allow them to come together in a way that helps maintain the shape of the breast. This is done after the pathologist has analyzed the lumpectomy specimen and feels the edges of the specimen are clear of tumor. The back edges of the breast can be allowed to come together naturally or can be sutured together with absorbable sutures. In essence, flap advancement is an uncomplicated way of helping to fill the cavity left by the lump removal, but it requires an artistic touch to be truly effective. The best skin closures are those that incorporate meticulous subcuticular plastic surgical techniques that leave no puckering or "railroad tracks" on the breast. Some surgeons use staples or "baseball" closures, stitching under and over the incision line. Baseball stitches can create scarring outside the incision line. I close the incision underneath the skin with a fine subcuticular closure so that the sutures are only visible at the ends of the incision.

I'll talk more about surgical options and flap advancement in Chapter 6, "Saving the Breast," but I want to point out that not every surgeon is familiar and facile with these techniques. If you are concerned about the appearance of your breast after excisional biopsy or breast saving surgery for breast cancer, request to see photographs of some of the surgeon's patients, ask how the incision will be made and closed and how you will look afterwards. I can't state often enough how important it is to make sure you are in the hands of a surgeon who performs breast cancer surgery as a major part of his or her practice. A surgeon's expertise and artistic ability can make all the difference in the way your breast looks after surgery and can also influence the type of surgery you will ultimately receive should your lump be malignant.

What Will You Do if the Lump Is Malignant?

It's important to realize that even the most benign-looking lump could be malignant. And while it's very difficult to contemplate the possibility of a cancer diagnosis, cancer is treatable, especially if found early. Although it is always possible for a cancer to spread before it's detected, the earlier it is diagnosed and treated, the better the likelihood that the cancer can be controlled.

Before you plan an open biopsy (surgical removal of a breast lump), you and your surgeon should discuss the results of your needle biopsies and any X-ray studies that you've had, such as a mammogram or ultrasound. If, on the basis of this information, it appears that you have a suspicious abnormality, you and your surgeon should discuss breast saving surgery for breast cancer, including the possibility of a larger lumpectomy and sentinel node mapping at the same time to potentially prevent the need for a second surgery. (Dr. Harlow discusses sentinel node biopsy in Chapter 8, "Removing Lymph Nodes." Sentinel node mapping is defined here as sentinel node biopsy with the removal of additional nearby lymph nodes.) Unless you have another illness that makes hospitalization necessary, the operation will be done in an outpatient setting while you are under general anesthesia. If you elect to avoid any type of preoperative needle biopsy and simply have the lump removed, you can still be made aware of the possibility of breast saving surgery and sentinel node mapping at the time of open biopsy, which is based on the frozen section diagnosis during surgery. Core needle biopsy with frozen section can occasionally be performed as the initial maneuver after you are under anesthesia to get a definitive diagnosis. Frozen section diagnosis is a rapid microscopic evaluation of the area surgically removed from your breast. The pathologist, who should be in the operating room at the time of your surgery, performs the frozen section by freezing a tiny bit of tissue to look at under the microscope in order to give the surgeon immediate information about the malignant or benign nature of the area removed. Frozen section diagnosis also helps us determine, if there is a malignancy, whether we got all of the cancer out with a healthy margin of normal tissue around it.

The use of frozen section depends a great deal on the expertise and experience of the pathologist. An excellent, experienced pathologist can perform frozen section for solid masses very well, whereas a less experienced pathologist might have more difficulty. You may want to ask your surgeon how experienced the pathologist is at breast pathology and if he or she will analyze the lump microscopically while you are in surgery. If you are in a situation in which a very experienced pathologist is unavailable, you will absolutely want to have a core needle biopsy done a week or so before your surgery so that you will know whether your lump is malignant or benign before surgery.

Permanent section, which involves a thorough analysis of the specimen, will provide the final results and will be available in a day or two following surgery. It's very important to understand that until the final pathology results are in, we will not know for certain whether we have removed all of the cancer with an adequate margin of clearance. I talk about breast saving surgery, including lumpectomy, and the concept of getting clear margins in Chapter 6, "Saving the Breast." If we do not get clear margins, more surgery will be necessary to get a clear margin and help prevent a recurrence of cancer in this area of the breast. You may also want to take a look at Chapter 8, "Removing Lymph Nodes," to gain a basic understanding of sentinel node biopsy.

Mastectomy is not done at the time of open biopsy in my practice. When planning an open biopsy, do not request that the surgeon decide whether to do a mastectomy at the time of biopsy, if the diagnosis is positive for cancer. You will need time to think about and absorb the possibility of mastectomy. Your thoughts and feelings about the loss of your breast may change. Likewise, you may decide to have an immediate breast reconstruction, which changes the way your mastectomy should be done. You may also want time to get a second opinion after your biopsy.

Cancer is not a death sentence. I've learned a lot about myself and about others through cancer. I've met a lot of people who I now consider my good friends. It's important to be positive. Of course I went through all the usual tears, but laughter helped me through it. I feel proud of myself that I made it. · Linda R.

When you're first diagnosed, the news that you have cancer can be overwhelming. You may feel anxious or panicky, and you may not comprehend all the information you're given. It's okay to ask about antianxiety medication. You might feel more comfortable and be able to absorb more information. · Joelle

What an incredible spiritual wake-up call. . . . I know that God has a reason for all things, and many times we won't become aware of them on earth. It's important to know that cancer is not a death sentence and that there is light at the end of the tunnel. · Linda L.

I came with a list of questions already knowing it was bad news. Two days earlier, I had a mammogram, which was followed by two more sets of pictures, an ultrasound, and a biopsy. That was one of the few days I broke down and cried for what seemed like hours, alone in my car in the parking lot. I still don't remember the drive home. · Cynthia

Too often we feel cancer equals death. But cancer does not equal death. I had a lot of faith, probably from my Irish-Catholic background. My mother used to repeat the old adage, "God doesn't close a door without opening a window," which greatly sustained me. I've gotten a lot of insight into myself as a result of my cancer diagnosis. In truth, I'm a better person than before I had breast cancer. A positive outlook has a lot to do with your eventual recovery. I never thought I wasn't going to survive. I have four kids and I know I'm going to be around to drive them crazy.
· Ann

BREAST CANCER AND BREAST LUMPS IN MEN

One percent of all breast cancers occur in men. Although the overwhelming majority of breast lumps in men are not cancerous, breast lumps in men should be taken seriously. Breast cancer in men is a virulent disease. A man who feels a lump in his breast should seek the attention of an appropriate physician, and diagnosis of a breast lump should never be delayed. Breast cancer is not an insult to one's manhood, nor is it related to any feminine characteristics.

Most lumps in men are due to some form of gynecomastia, or male breast enlargement, which is a benign condition and a very common problem. This typically occurs in men in their teens and twenties or men in their fifties or sixties. Gynecomastia can occur naturally or can be brought on by male steroid use, excessive alcohol intake, liver disease, and certain medications and can occur in one or both breasts as a firm mass or as a diffuse enlargement of the male breast. A complete history and physical examination is helpful to look for potential causes of gynecomastia.

When gynecomastia occurs as a firm lump, I frequently perform fine needle aspiration to check for suspicious or malignant cells in men above the age of 30. Mammography can also be used as a diagnostic tool to evaluate firm masses in men, and all relevant lymph node areas should be checked thoroughly. When all diagnostic information indicates that a breast mass is gynecomastia, you have the option of a cosmetic removal of the gynecomastia, depending on how much it bothers you. This requires the removal of the male breast through a small periareolar incision performed as an outpatient surgical procedure under general anesthetic. No significant deformity generally results and, in expert hands, no reconstructive maneuvers are required. Gynecomastia can grow and become unsightly, and most men with significant gynecomastia want it surgically corrected.

Breast masses that are suspicious for breast cancer should be approached differently from masses likely to be gynecomastia. Preoperative fine needle aspiration or core needle biopsies will likely reveal the malignant nature of these tumors and should lead to a discussion of modified radical mastectomy in a man. Breast saving surgery is not an option for male breast cancer due to the small size of the male breast and the virulence of the disease. Evaluation by a medical oncologist is warranted preoperatively if any suggestion of disease spread is evident on physical examination, chest X-ray, or preoperative lab work. Otherwise, a medical oncologist will evaluate you after surgery for staging and a discussion of chemotherapy and/or radiation. Men and their physicians should never ignore a firm breast mass in a man because they think that breast cancer can't occur in men. If you are a man with a firm breast mass, make sure that you come away from your interaction with your physician with a definitive diagnosis. Again, this requires some type of tissue diagnosis obtained by a needle biopsy or a surgical biopsy.

CHAPTER TWO

You've Just Been Told That You Have an Abnormal Mammogram

By Daniel Kirsch, M.D.

If there is a finding on your routine screening mammogram, or you or your physician suspect that you have a breast lump, it's likely that you will have additional imaging tests to further characterize the abnormality to determine the most appropriate work-up. Your radiologist may use additional mammographic views, sonography, or magnetic resonance imaging (MRI) to accomplish this task.

Having a Diagnostic Mammogram

The two most common diagnostic mammographic views are magnification and spot compression. Magnification is used to better visualize the small calcifications that are sometimes seen on mammograms. Small calcifications can indicate malignancy, such as in situ carcinoma (cancer that has not yet traveled outside the milk ducts). They can be so small as to be barely visible, much less characterizable by their morphology (shape) and distribution, two features that are important in determining whether they should be biopsied. Magnification views position the

A *radiologist* is a physician who is trained to diagnose disease using imaging studies, such as mammograms, ultrasound, CT, and MRI. A *breast imaging radiologist* detects breast cancer through imaging techniques and is adept at performing needle biopsies, which demand a high level of expertise and skill.

calcifications farther away from the film to enlarge their images and make them easier to evaluate. Spot compression views are usually performed to further assess a mammographically detected mass or focal density (an area of density that does not meet strict criteria for a mass but might have the potential to be a mass). A smaller than standard compression paddle is used for this technique. It is placed directly over the area of interest, allowing for better visualization of the lesion or suspected lesion. Often, what was initially suspected as a possible abnormality presses or "squishes" out, effectively disappearing, and requiring no further evaluation. At other times, this technique not only confirms that a true lesion is present—perhaps one that was only a subtle area of asymmetric density on the standard screening study—but renders its details suspicious for malignancy.

Breast Ultrasound

Breast ultrasound, or sonography, is a powerful tool used frequently in the diagnosis of breast disease. Most simply, it is used to determine if a mammographic or palpable mass (a lump that can be felt) is a cyst or a solid lesion. Many times, the solid or cystic nature of a mass can be inferred from the way it looks on your mammogram, but it can't be determined with certainty as it can on an ultrasound. The distinction between solid and cystic lesions is important: simple cysts (cysts filled with fluid only) are benign and, in the absence of associated symptoms, may be left alone without risk of cancer developing. Radiologists are sometimes asked to aspirate these cysts using ultrasound guidance. This is usually a quick, simple pro-

WHAT IS BREAST ULTRASOUND?

Breast ultrasound utilizes the interaction between short pulses of high-frequency sound energy with tissue to generate an electronic two-dimensional display of the breast.

cedure, but one that is indicated only when the cyst is causing pain or discomfort, is enlarging, or is otherwise bothersome. Complex cysts— that is, cysts with solid material inside or material attached to the walls—may require biopsy or excision.

If an ultrasound shows a mass to be solid, a biopsy is usually indicated. The high-resolution sonography available today allows for detailed inspection of a lesion's features. Close characterization of its shape, echotexture (brightness), margins, and size can predict with reasonable accuracy the likelihood of benignancy or malignancy but not, as of yet, to the standards required for accepted patient care. Therefore, we are often obligated to biopsy a lesion that we can comfortably state has an 80 to 90 percent chance of being benign. Much of the anxiety associated with biopsy could be alleviated if this information were to be communicated to patients before the procedure.

> ## MOST BREAST LESIONS ARE BENIGN
>
> Ultrasound can determine whether a mass is cystic or solid and can help predict whether a lesion is malignant or benign, but because ultrasound can't determine whether a solid mass is malignant or benign with absolute certainty, a biopsy may be indicated even when a lump is very likely not to be cancerous.

Although breast ultrasound is a powerful tool, it is not generally appropriate as a screening procedure. Both patients and physicians frequently misunderstand this. Breast ultrasound is best performed in a *directed* fashion to target as specific an area as possible, usually a single quadrant of the breast. For instance, if a mass is detected by mammography at the "ten o'clock position of the left breast," detailed and directed ultrasound scanning of the upper inner quadrant of the left breast is undertaken. Many times a correlative lesion (a lesion that corresponds to the mammogram at ultrasound) is identified only after exhaustive and careful inspection, even when the region being evaluated is small. Scanning the entire breast, much less both breasts, to the same exactness is tremendously time-consuming. Although some people report a modicum of success with this technique, it must be considered impractical at this time. Generally, it's best to think of breast ultrasound as appropriate for further evaluation of palpable masses and those identified by mammography.

Magnetic Resonance Imaging (MRI)

MRI is used much less frequently than ultrasound and diagnostic breast imaging. It can, however, be quite useful in certain clinical scenarios and possesses tremendous potential. Some radiologists believe that MRI will eventually replace mammography for both screening and diagnostic purposes. Indeed, MRI has enviable sensitivity; that is, it is extremely able to detect disease when present. But it may be too sensitive. With MRI, it's sometimes difficult to distinguish between disease and normal breast tissue, much less between benign and malignant processes. With more experience and further technical developments, this will likely be overcome. Currently, this problem can lead to many unnecessary biopsies, resulting in significant cost both in terms of dollars and cents and with respect to patient anxiety. There is another problem with MRI. Sometimes a lesion/lump can only be seen on an MRI and isn't identified/located by mammography, ultrasound, or physical examination. In such cases, biopsy becomes a difficult matter. As will be discussed later in this chapter, most breast lesions are biopsied by mammographic or sonographic guidance and, if lumpectomy is necessary, localized (identified) for the surgeon using wires by these methods. MRI-guided localizations and biopsy are highly specialized procedures, performed at very few institutions, usually large teaching and research centers. Even at such places, these techniques are not commonplace and are often difficult. The result can be a suspicious finding that is seen only by MRI with no straightforward way to get it out.

MRI is also very expensive. If it is to be used in a widespread manner, it will have to be made much more affordable. For the time being, MRI is usually used in special circumstances, including patients in whom there is an equivocal mammographic finding, a personal or family history of breast cancer, and patients with malignant axillary lymph nodes and no mammographic evidence of cancer.

| DIGITAL MAMMOGRAPHY

In the field of radiology, contrast resolution refers to the ability to differentiate shades of gray. A cancer surrounded by fatty tissue is conspicuous on film because its density is quite different than the more transparent fat. Thus, the contrast is quite high. When a cancer is surrounded by tissue of similar density, such as glandular tissue, the contrast is reduced, and cancer becomes much more difficult to detect. Our ability to differentiate between normal and abnormal tissue is further hindered by a fundamental property of X-ray film. When properly exposed, the region of film on which glandular tissues are recorded has lower inherent contrast than the region of film on which fatty tissues are captured. As a result, masses surrounded by glandular tissue are imaged at a lower contrast than those superimposed with adjacent fat. This "low contrast detection" is a fundamental limitation of standard film-screen mammography. This is why mammography can be difficult for dense breasts and the primary reason for the interest in developing other methods of recording the diagnostic information.

Digital image receptors, developed to substitute for the standard film-screen receptor, are one such method. *Digital* simply means that the picture is comprised of and divided into rows and columns made of up of smaller blocks called pixels whose gray scale—that is, how light and dark they are—is defined by numbers. A number is assigned to each individual pixel and that number defines its specific shade of gray. When the pixels are viewed together, an image is produced. There are numerous practical advantages to this system. Because the image is essentially a collection of numbers, it can be reproduced over and over without loss of information. It can also be manipulated. For example, it can be made lighter or darker or bigger or smaller. It can be electronically stored and can be transmitted (as a series of numbers) over wires and cables. It can also be subjected to various computer analyses that might aid in overall interpretation. All of this means, for instance, that in a matter of minutes or seconds your study could be sent electronically to a location far from where it was performed to be interpreted, say, by an expert mammographer who is aided in the diagnostic process by a computer program that can highlight or "tag" calcifications or areas of perceived increased or asymmetric density. This is called *teleconsultation* and *computer-aided detection*.

Because digital images can be displayed differently from the way in which they were

> ### FINDING DIGITAL MAMMOGRAPHY CAN BE DIFFICULT
>
> At the time of this writing, few institutions have digital mammography systems, although you would most likely find them in major academic institutions.

DIGITAL MAMMOGRAPHY

(*Continued*)

acquired—that is, they can be shown as lighter or darker, or from different angles and obliquities—they are likely to improve contrast between tissues and aid in cancer detection overall. Of course, digital mammography is not without its limitations. Modern mammography requires high spatial resolution (*spatial resolution* refers to the smallness at which an entity can be viewed before it can no longer be seen as discreet), and achieving this has been a problem for digital systems. If we are to avoid film and its limitations, we must have another way of viewing the image. This has been accomplished with high-resolution monitors—video screens, if you will. But even these high-resolution monitors have been unable to provide all the information needed to an exacting degree. Improvements in display technology continue, however, and more and more digital systems are coming into clinical use. In fact, we are at a point at which the cost involved in setting up such a system, rather than the actual current technical limitations, is impeding digital mammography's overall implementation.

Breast Intervention: Getting a Diagnosis without Surgery

The past several years have seen a dramatic change in the way most breast lesions are evaluated. If, for example, you were told that your mammogram showed a mass or group of calcifications, traditionally you would have had surgery called an *excisional* or *open biopsy* in which a surgeon removed the lesion.

Surgery of this type is not always ideal for a number of reasons. First, there is a substantial difference between the kind of surgical procedure performed to obtain a diagnosis and that required to *treat* a known cancer. A simple biopsy usually requires only a small incision and removal of minimal breast tissue. A lumpectomy removes more tissue, necessitates a bigger incision, and may require accompanying reconstructive surgery and lymph node removal. With a traditional work-up, you would not know which of these different procedures was necessary. You would not know beforehand whether the lesion found by mammography was benign or malignant and hence whether you were about to undergo a minimal surgery or potentially longer operation.

The traditional scenario also requires the pathologist to perform what is referred to as a *frozen section.* The surgical specimen (or part of it) is frozen so that the pathologist can render an on-the-spot interpretation of the benign or malignant nature of the tumor or calcifications while you are on the operating table under anesthesia. Depending on the experience and expertise of the pathologist, frozen section diagnosis can be difficult, especially for calcifications.

Most lesions biopsied in the breast are benign. Benign findings occur, in essence, because mammography is a screening test performed on asymptomatic people to detect breast cancer before signs and symptoms develop. But mammograms have limitations, including false positives and false negatives. A false positive is when the test indicates the presence of disease when there isn't any. A false negative is when the test indicates that there is no disease when, in fact, there is.

Every day mammograms read as suspicious or possibly suspicious for cancer result in biopsies that turn out to be benign. In fact, 70 to 80 percent of properly indicated breast biopsies turn out to be benign, which means thousands of surgeries for benign disease. Some women want *any* lesion excised, but if we could identify the benign lesion before the surgical stage, most of these surgeries could be avoided. In fact, for the most part, we can. With few exceptions, we can obtain diagnosis of a mammographically or sonographically detected lesion without surgery. Patients must understand that with benign needle biopsies, the lesion is not removed. It will continue to appear on subsequent films and must be observed for any future growth.

Detection happens when we biopsy the lesion in a minimally invasive fashion with a needle. There are two types of needle biopsies: core and fine needle aspiration. Core biopsies are performed with a large-gauge (usually 14–11 gauge) needle that, by virtue of a notchlike defect near the tip of the needle, shears off a sliver or core of tissue from the area of concern. There are actually two needles in such a system: an inner needle, containing the notch, and an outer, cutting needle that advances a fraction of a second after the inner needle is deployed, or "fired," covering it like a tight sleeve. When the outer needle passes over the notch defect in the inner one, tissue is compressed into the opening and sheared, producing specimens that are actually strings of tissue. Core biopsies can be performed by stereotactic guidance (see below) or ultrasound guidance and therefore are used to biopsy both masses and calcifications.

Fine needle biopsies are performed with small-gauge (usually 25–21 gauge) "skinny" needles. These are usually done by ultrasound (or palpation) guidance and are generally limited to biopsy of masses. With this technique, only scant amounts of tissue are obtained. To evaluate the minute specimens requires pathologic expertise in cytology—a relative rarity in the United States—as well as competence in the actual physical technique of the procedure itself, a skill deceptively difficult to master and one that is often not appreciated by physicians performing them. These two requirements have limited the use of this type of biopsy in this country, accounting for the unfortunate and not infrequent result of "insufficient tissue for diagnosis" on pathology reports. Nonetheless, with the proper personnel, it is an extremely useful and accurate procedure and is certainly the most minimally invasive method of obtaining a tissue diagnosis.

Core biopsies are more straightforward to evaluate. The pathologist is able to evaluate the tissue as a whole and need not be an expert in cytopathology where the evaluation of individual cells is required. These biopsies are performed by ultrasound or stereotactic guidance, and therefore, as previously stated, can be used to biopsy masses or calcifications. For success, ultrasound guidance requires eye-hand coordination and experience—it is an acquired skill. Its concept, however, is simple: direct observation by ultrasound of the needle within the breast to place it into the target to obtain tissue. There is visual confirmation of the needle in the lesion. This is then documented on film or videotape. Some solid masses can be difficult to needle biopsy by ultrasound guidance. When this occurs, it is generally because of their specific location within the breast. In such cases, excision may be necessary.

Stereotactic Guidance

Stereotactic guidance is essentially X-ray or mammographic guidance of needle biopsy, but with a third dimension. By obtaining X-rays at 30 degrees from one another, and using something called *parallax shift* (actually a simple geometric property), the computer triangulates the location of the lesion in the x, y, and z planes; in other words, in three dimensions. The stereotactic equipment then positions the biopsy device so that tissue can be obtained. Whatever the finding on the mammogram—be it mass or calcifications—it can, for the most part, be biopsied by this method. (There are, of course, exceptions. Sometimes, stereotactic biopsy may not be possible in very small breasts, and sometimes the location of the lesion within the breast renders it inaccessible.) The machine's ability to place the probe accurately is quite remarkable and has made reliable biopsy of truly tiny clusters of calcifications routine.

Mammotome

Directed vacuum-assisted biopsy, otherwise known as *Mammotome core biopsy,* is a relatively new technology. Originally developed for use with stereotactic machines, it is now available for use with ultrasound as well and has proven to be a significant advance in needle biopsy technology. With these devices, the needle positioned in the breast is hollow and attached to a vacuum canister. Once in position, the vacuum draws tissue into a side hole in the needle. A rotating cutter then passes through the hollow needle, cuts a piece or core of the tissue, and sucks it through the needle, where it is collected in a chamber outside the breast.

There are several advantages to this biopsy method. Foremost, the volume of tissue obtained is considerably greater than with the traditional core biopsy "gun." Mammotome biopsies are usually done with 11-gauge needles (although 14-gauge needles have also been available), yielding specimens that are almost three times the size as each of those obtained with a standard 14-gauge gun-needle combination. Several studies have confirmed what intuition might have predicted: The larger volume of specimen translates into greater biopsy success. This is particularly true for the biopsy of calcifications. The biopsy of calcifications, which can be quite difficult with traditional needle-gun systems, is rarely a problem with 11-gauge vacuum-assisted biopsy. In experienced hands, success has been documented in more than 95 percent of cases. There is a high likelihood of getting a definitive diagnosis with this method. The larger specimens also aid in differentiating between lesions that can be challenging to define pathologically. Chief among these is distinguishing ductal carcinoma in situ (DCIS) from atypical hyperplasia (tissue that is not malignant but is abnormal and carries an increased risk of malignancy), and to a lesser degree, invasive from in situ carcinoma. For more information on DCIS, see Chapter 10, "Chemotherapy, Hormone Therapy, and the Stages of Breast Cancer."

Unlike conventional needle-gun systems, vacuum-assisted biopsy doesn't require removal of the needle each time a sample is taken. Once the needle is in place within the breast, it is not removed until after all the biopsy material has been obtained. The procedure is quicker, less cumbersome, and generally less traumatic to the breast. The Mammotome system allows the needle to be "dialed" to the desired position within the breast and does not require using the spring-loaded firing mechanism that needle-gun systems are dependent upon. The advantage of this is a reduction in the minimum breast thickness required for stereotactic biopsy, potentially allowing biopsy of smaller breasts. Traditional spring-loaded systems cannot be used to biopsy very small breasts because of the risk of the needle going through the entire breast. This risk is eliminated with the Mammotome system.

Despite the large samples yielded by core biopsy, it is an extremely safe and generally well-tolerated procedure. Significant complications are extremely rare (one study reported a 0.2 percent rate in over 3,700 biopsies[1]) and usually confined to infection and hematoma, both of which are readily treatable. Mild post-procedure pain and bruising have been reported to occur in about one-third of patients. Patients are instructed to stop taking aspirin and other nonsteroidal anti-inflammatory drugs (NSAIDS), such as Motrin or Advil, three days prior to the biopsy to minimize the risk of procedure-related bleeding.

---

[1] Parker, S.H., Burbank, F., Jackman, R.J., et al. "Percutaneous large core biopsy: a multi-institutional study." *Journal of Radiology,* 1994, Nov, 193(2): 359–64.

Having a Core Needle Biopsy by Stereotactic or Ultrasound Guidance

Before a core needle biopsy, a local anesthetic is injected just under the skin of the area to be biopsied. A small incision (about a quarter of an inch) is required for both stereotactic or ultrasound-guided core needle biopsies. Once started, the entire process is usually completed in 15 to 30 minutes. Biopsy of calcifications usually takes slightly longer than for masses, because an additional X ray is done in order to prove a successful retrieval of the calcifications. Steri-strip bandages are placed over the incision after the biopsy. No sutures (stitches) are required. Use of an ice pack over the biopsy site for several hours is generally advocated.

Not surprisingly, stress is the most prevalent complication associated with core needle biopsy. In one study, 50 percent of women described the stress they experienced as debilitating for up to 24 hours following biopsy, preventing them from resuming normal activities during that time.[2] This undoubtedly has to do with the anticipation of the biopsy result. Some women may also experience stress before the procedure. Taking an anxiolytic (such as low-dose Xanax or Valium) shortly before the biopsy can help reduce stress around the time of biopsy, although in my practice the most common comment I hear from patients after a core needle biopsy is, "That wasn't as bad as I thought it would be."

Wire Localization

Once a lesion is determined to be malignant or pre-malignant, surgical excision is required. How is a mass or group of calcifications that is seen only by mammography or ultrasound (a nonpalpable mass) surgically removed? How does the surgeon know where it is? If you were to see the breast as a surgeon does in the operating room, you would see a

---

[2] Derhsaw, D.D., Karavalla, B.A., "Limitations and complications in the utilization of stereotactic core breast biopsies." *Breast Journal*, 1996, v. 2: 13–17.

mound of yellow tissue with essentially no landmarks to indicate where you are. The guide for surgeons is a procedure called *wire localization.* After a local anesthetic and a sterile prep, one or more wires are placed into the breast through the skin, terminating adjacent to or within the area of concern. During your operation, the surgeon will dissect along the wire from the skin until he or she reaches the distal portion of the wire, usually indicated by a thickening or a hook, which should then reveal the sought-after lesion. The wires can be placed by one of three guidance methods: conventional mammography in which you are seated as for a routine mammographic exam, or by stereotactic or ultrasound guidance. The modality that most clearly depicts the abnormality is usually the most appropriate one to use.

The idea behind wire localization is the same as for biopsies guided by these methods, except that a localization needle is placed into the targeted area instead of a biopsy needle. Once the desired position is confirmed, a smaller and very skinny wire is threaded through the needle, and the needle is removed. You will leave the radiology suite with the wire in your breast, poking out through the skin, although it is usually taped gently against the chest wall and covered by a gauze pad.

Some surgeons find bracketing wire localization very advantageous. *Bracketing* means that two, or sometimes more, wires are placed so that they encompass the lesion, defining two or more of its margins. This method was originally used to indicate the extent of a very large or poorly defined group of calcifications when their extent could not be indicated by one wire alone.

With improving surgical techniques, the goal of removing as little tissue as possible without compromising the surgery's therapeutic success has become realistic. Bracketing localizations can be quite helpful here. Wires situated along the margins of the tumor allow the surgeon to sculpt around the mass or cluster of calcifications, removing it intact with an appropriate amount of surrounding breast tissue, without directly encountering it. Avoiding violation of the tumor-breast interface by this technique is something that has at least theoretical advantage for overall outcome in breast cancer surgery. This bracketing wire technique can also be quite useful when a benign or a suspected benign lesion is being removed and a primary concern is the concomitant removal of as little normal tissue as possible.

Localization is an odd experience. They put you in the mammogram machine and take an X ray to find the calcifications. They then put a needle in the middle of that area or bracket it with needles on two sides so the surgeon knows where to biopsy. After the needle is placed, they take another picture to make sure it's in the right place and move the needle if it's not. It hurts, but not terribly. It's more the act of sitting there and looking at yourself with this big old needle sticking out of you that's so strange. • Joelle

You're having a mammogram and at the same they are trying to localize the mass to determine where to cut. It's not a comfortable procedure, but I must say all the technicians were right there for me. They were very kind and very sensitive to what was happening. • Linda L.

Although very uncomfortable, the procedure was interesting. The radiologist would take more mammogram pictures and insert the needles around the area that needed to be removed. Somehow, I felt better having seen this and much more confident that they would be able to remove all of the cancer. • Cynthia

Is Your Biopsy Accurate? What You Need to Know about "The Triple Test."

Perhaps the most important information to take away from this chapter is the concept of imaging-pathology correlation. On the surface, biopsy appears quite simple: there is a lesion in the breast, biopsy is performed, and the diagnosis is obtained. Unfortunately, the reality isn't this straightforward. First, what appears to be a lesion by imaging or palpation isn't always a lesion. Normal breast tissue can appear abnormal, usually focally prominent or asymmetric when compared to the opposite breast and can be interpreted as a suspicious lesion when in fact it isn't one at all.

Problems can also occur with the biopsy. This usually has to do with what we call *sampling error.* Simply, the lesion was missed. The needle may be right around the lesion or may be within it, but the samples obtained are not representative of its true pathology. Occasionally, and particularly in less experienced hands, something is misinterpreted at biopsy as a suspicious lesion when it is really something else, and the true lesion is never biopsied.

Rarely, the pathologist can make a mistake on a core needle biopsy. The distinction between cancer and "not cancer" isn't always as clear as it seems it should be. Distinguishing between simply benign and atypical lesions is even more difficult. Atypical lesions carry an increased risk of subsequent frank malignancy and are therefore removed surgically, whereas no further action is usually required for simply benign lesions.

If this is unsettling, it should be. Most people don't think to question their needle biopsy results, and many primary care physicians fail to realize how important this concept is. The bottom line is: *The results of the needle biopsy must be consistent with the findings on the mammogram or ultrasound.* Radiologists refer to this as *concordance* and *discordance.* We also use the term *triple test,* meaning that in order to be satisfied that a work-up of a suspected lesion is complete and accurate, the findings on the clinical breast exam, mammography or ultrasound, and biopsy must all be consistent with one another. If any are not, there is a risk that cancer could be missed.

For example, say you are told that your mammogram showed a small mass with irregular features, which was new from your prior mammogram. Your clinical breast exam is normal, but a correlative ultrasound shows a solid mass in the location of the mammographic finding. A biopsy is therefore recommended, and you choose to have this done as a core biopsy with ultrasound (or stereotactic) guidance. Of course, you are very relieved when your doctor calls you to report that the biopsy was negative, or benign. Your emotions are quite different, however, when you are told at your next mammogram one year later that the mass is bigger, needs to be biopsied once again, and, in fact, is determined to be malignant.

What happened? Upon closer review of the *initial* biopsy report, one finds that what was described was simply normal breast tissue. True, there was no evidence of malignancy but there was nothing other than normal breast tissue. This is a discordant result. The finding of normal breast tissue on the biopsy does not match the mammogram and ultrasound findings, which showed a true, though small, mass. In order for us to accept the biopsy result, we need to have something that is consistent with an actual mass, be it malignant or benign. In this case, the mass was missed on the biopsy and only the surrounding breast tissue was actually sampled. The failure of the triple test should have been recognized and prompted repeat biopsy, possibly by excision at this point.

It should be pointed out that the same logic and potential for error exists with surgical biopsies, although this can be largely alleviated with the use of careful specimen imaging. A radiograph (X ray) or sonogram of the actual excised breast specimen is performed to ensure that it contains the lesion or area of concern. Whatever the method of final diagnosis, consistency between clinical evaluation, imaging findings, and biopsy results must be established.

You don't need to be a physician to be your own advocate, and you don't need a deep understanding of all the related terminology and principles. If you have had a biopsy, ask your doctors, including your radiologist, whether the biopsy result makes sense for the mammographic and sonographic findings that prompted the biopsy in the first place. No one should be comfortable until the triple test is fulfilled.

My tumor was caught on a mammogram. I had no clue that I had cancer and no discomfort, so when the radiologist came in and said, "We have a problem," it was as if someone had thrown a bucket of water on my face. I thought he was going to say what he always said, which was, "See you next year." • Beverly

I started having mammograms every year. I had a clean mammogram the November before I discovered my lump. The type of cancer I had was very aggressive and very fast growing. If you feel a lump, even if you've had a mammogram, get it checked out. Most of the time it may not be anything, but it could be. • Anne

Screening Mammography

Mammography is unique among medical tests, certainly among imaging procedures, because it's done for one purpose only: to detect cancer. Screening mammography is done for asymptomatic women—women who have no signs or symptoms of breast cancer—to detect the disease at a smaller size and stage than it would be diagnosed otherwise. There is intuitive sense in the notion that the smaller a breast cancer is when detected and the sooner it is treated, the less likely it is to have metastasized (spread), and the greater the chance that the patient can be cured. This is the basic tenet supporting the use of screening mammography. If you have followed reports of the studies over the past ten years in the popular press, however, you will know that the question of whether this is true or not is quite controversial.

There have been more than ten major national and international studies over the past ten years designed to determine if screening mammography works; that is, if it decreases mortality and by how much. The fact that there have been so many studies, as well as numerous commentaries and epidemiological analyses is a testament to the controversy. Roughly half of these studies demonstrate success and half do not. To those of us who believe in screening, there are clear explanations accounting for the unfavorable studies. Without going into detail, these include poor quality mammograms, use of untrained interpreters, and flawed study designs.

To be sure, there are legitimate issues with respect to the potential problems with screening. Some investigators credit decreased mortality more to the improved treatment of breast cancer than to early detection. Many critics of screening cite the well-known epidemiological concepts of *lead-* and *length-time bias.* An in-depth discussion of these concepts is beyond the scope of this chapter, but generally, lead-time bias refers to the phenomenon that earlier diagnosis does not in and of itself mean that a patient will live longer, it may merely increase the time that she knows she has cancer. Length-time bias suggests that less aggressive, slower-growing tumors (with inherently better prognoses) are primarily detected by mammograms, while the faster growing, more lethal tumors are often found clinically.

The most recent major study at the time of this writing that supports the effectiveness of mammography screening is authored by well-known breast imaging expert László Tabár, and published in May 2001 in the journal *Cancer.* He found that among 6,807 Swedish women followed over a 29-year period, there was a 63 percent reduction in breast cancer deaths among those who were actually screened.

This is about twice the benefit commonly reported, even in past favorable studies.

As the controversy is played out, the words of two other breast imaging experts may summarize the issue:

> We support the routine use of mammographic screening . . . because we interpret the evidence as indicating a high probability of benefit. It seems much more prudent to endorse screening now and risk the unlikely subsequent determination that the effort was ineffective, than to withhold screening until it is determined whether "proof" will be obtained and risk the loss of so many women in the prime of life. . . . The decision to screen represents an opportunity for—not a guarantee of—early detection and diagnosis, but the decision not to screen represents the loss of this opportunity.[3]

There are four exposures taken during screening mammography, two for each breast. The standard views are termed *cranicocaudad* (CC) and *mediolateral oblique* (MLD) and essentially image each breast from the top down and sideways. A slighty skewed view is used to include more breast tissue in the field. The MLO views tend to include more overall tissue while the CC views are usually more reproducible with respect to positioning.

Each time a woman or man has a mammogram she or he will receive a dose of approximately 0.1 rad per breast, although this will vary depending on breast thickness and density, among other factors. There is miniscule theoretical risk of inducing malignancy in the screening population over the age of 40 years at the present levels of radiation exposure. There are, however, times when it is wise to avoid radiation exposure. Women under age 30 and those who are pregnant or lactating should avoid screening studies, as these are times when the breast tissue is most biologically active and most vulnerable to the deleterious effects of ionizing radiation.

Many women don't like the compression required for mammography, but taut compression is essential for high-quality images that

---

[3] Sickles, E., Kopans, D. 1995. *Annals of Internal Medicine,* quoted in L. Berlin, "Dot Size, Lead Time, Fallibility, and Impact on Survival," Berlin, L. *AJR,* May 2001: 176.

enable diagnosis of very small and early lesions. Compression spreads out information; it evens out tissues from the chest wall to the nipple so both thick and thin portions can be viewed. It brings objects closer to the film, improving their resolution. It holds the breast still, preventing motion and image blurring. It also reduces breast thickness, lowering the required radiation dose, and thins out the breast tissue, reducing X-ray scatter. Compression may be unpleasant for a brief period of time, but it's probably the single most important factor in determining whether an optimal study will be achieved, and all efforts within reason should be made to apply and withstand it.

In Summary: Points to Remember

• Begin your routine mammographic screening at the age of 40, preferably at a center with a specialty-trained mammographer.

• If you have an abnormality on your mammogram or ultrasound that cannot be felt by an experienced physician, discuss the possibility of image-guided needle biopsy with your primary care physician or breast surgeon. Do not hesitate to include the breast imager (radiologist) in this discussion.

• If you elect an image-guided needle biopsy, make sure that the results of the biopsy match the appearance of the abnormality on the original mammogram or ultrasound.

• If you have had an open procedure in which breast tissue is surgically removed with the assistance of wire localization, make sure that the procedure includes a specimen radiograph in order to confirm that the lesion was removed.

❧

CHAPTER THREE

You've Just Discovered That You Have a Nipple Discharge

By Gregory Senofsky, M.D., F.A.C.S., F.S.S.O.

It's not unusual for women to have some nipple discharge, which is often noted as a discoloration on the bra. The appearance of a discharge can be alarming, but most of the time, it's due to a benign condition. For example, spontaneous clear, white, and green discharges are often due to fibrocystic changes, lactation, or cysts. Duct ectasia, a condition in which the ducts behind the nipple are dilated and inflamed, is another less common cause of discharge. While these discharges may not signal cancer, it's important to see your physician for evaluation. After a thorough discussion and examination, your physician may suggest a breast ultrasound and/or a mammogram, depending on your age and the result of the physical examination.

Natural remedies for fibrocystic breasts (see Chapter 1, pages 5–18) can also ameliorate pain and nipple discharge that happens as a result of a fibrocystic condition. Occasionally, surgical removal of a small portion of the breast tissue behind the nipple and areola (the dark area of skin surrounding your nipple) is necessary to treat a bothersome nipple discharge that seems to be benign. If you are lactating inappropriately—in other words, you've not recently had a baby—your doctor should order a blood test to check your prolactin level, especially if you are having headaches and visual changes, such as a narrowing of the visual field. Prolactin is a pituitary gland hormone that stimulates milk production. The presence of prolactin in your blood when you are not breast-feeding can signify a pituitary tumor. Your physician might order a MRI or CT scan of your brain to rule out the possibility of this very unusual situation.

If You Notice Brown or Bloody Discharge

Brown or bloody discharge is of more concern and should never be ignored. In most cases, these discharges are caused by benign tumors, or small polyps called *intraductal papillomas,* lining the milk ducts behind the nipple. But brown or bloody nipple discharge can also be caused by nipple trauma, or by breast cancer eroding into a duct.

If you have brown or bloody discharge, see a breast specialist. Your doctor may refer you to a breast surgeon (see Chapter 19, "How to Get the Best Care and Treatment," for information on finding and choosing doctors who specialize in addressing breast concerns). Your breast surgeon should take a thorough history and do a physical examination, including an examination of your breast to see if the discharge is coming from one or many ducts. Pathologic assessment of the discharging fluid is often performed, but this is rarely helpful. If there is any question that the discharge contains blood, a hemocult test can be ordered to find out for certain if there is blood in the discharge. You should also have a mammogram and ultrasound. Before considering any surgery, you should have an X ray called a *ductogram.* This is a simple procedure performed by an experienced radiologist in which a tiny catheter is inserted into the duct through the nipple. A small amount of radiopaque dye is injected into the nipple while a mammogram is done. This allows us to see any growth or tumor behind the nipple. The ductogram can be a bit uncomfortable, but it doesn't usually hurt, and it won't affect the feeling in your nipple afterwards.

After your ductogram, you and your doctor must decide whether or not to remove the abnormal duct. Central duct excision is a minor outpatient surgical procedure. The duct is removed through a small incision placed cosmetically on the edge of the areola or within the areolar skin. This is done while you are asleep with the assistance of a tiny sterile probe slipped through the discharging duct to guide the surgeon to

the duct in question. If your ductogram reveals a growth likely to be
responsible for the brown or bloody
discharge, central duct excision is
imperative to determine whether
the growth is benign or malignant.
If the ductogram is normal, the
decision to operate is based on all
the information at hand. Sometimes
a woman and her physician may
decide to delay this procedure for a
short period of time in order to see
if the discharge stops. A delay is
fine, providing that there is no
lump and no abnormality detected

Ductoscopy is a new method of looking into ducts with tiny scopes. It is currently being evaluated as a tool that may prove helpful in the management of abnormal nipple discharges and possibly ductal carcinoma in situ (DCIS). Ductoscopy is a spin-off of ductal lavage, a technique that allows the clinician to wash out breast ducts through the nipple to look for abnormal cells. Ductal lavage is also being looked at as a potential diagnostic tool in high-risk patients. Please refer to Chapter 4, "The Ductal Approach to Diagnosis and Treatment of Breast Cancer" for more information.

on the mammogram and ultrasound, and the discharge hasn't been present for long. If the discharge persists, central duct excision can be performed to stop the discharge. Often, a tiny benign papilloma is found on the pathology assessment.

If your ductogram is quite suspicious —in other words, if there is a high likelihood of a malignancy—you and your doctor should discuss breast-saving surgery for breast cancer with possible sentinel node mapping. There are a few options to follow at this time:

• You and your doctor may decide to do a directed mammogram ultrasound of the suspicious area. A needle biopsy of the area should be considered to determine the exact nature of the area prior to surgery, if ultrasound or mammogram shows a discrete abnormality. If the needle biopsy proves to be malignant, preoperative wire localization may be used to assist in performing a central lumpectomy.

• A central duct excision can be performed and sent for permanent pathological analysis in anticipation of a likely second surgery.

• A central duct excision can be widened to a central lumpectomy with possible sentinel node mapping, depending on the frozen section analysis. (See Chapter 12, "Behind the Microscope" for more information about frozen section.) Patients must be told that this could involve excision of the nipple or the nipple/areola complex, if malignancy is documented.

Chapter 6, "Saving the Breast" contains a discussion of breast-saving surgery for breast cancer, including lumpectomy and other breast-conserving procedures. Breast-saving surgery for cancer in the presence of a bloody nipple discharge coming from the cancer requires excision of the nipple in continuity with the appropriate duct or tumor, all with a clear margin, a concept that I will discuss further in that chapter.

If You Notice the Skin of Your Nipple Is Itchy and Scaling

Most itching and scaling conditions of the nipple and areola are benign conditions; however, Paget's disease is an unusual type of early breast cancer that involves the nipple. It looks like eczema but it can indicate a breast cancer underlying the nipple. To investigate possible Paget's disease, your breast surgeon may take a small wedge from the skin of your nipple and areola using local anesthetic. In most cases, people with Paget's disease can be treated with breast-saving surgery, such as an extended lumpectomy in which the nipple, areola, and some of the central portion of the breast are removed. It is extremely important to remove the cancer that may lie behind the nipple/areola complex. Likewise, any abnormalities seen on a mammogram or ultrasound in this area should be included in the specimen, and sentinel node mapping should be discussed preoperatively. Abnormalities that can't be felt by touch, such as an abnormality seen on a mammogram, can be bracketed with localization wires placed in

BREAST-SAVING SURGERIES TO TREAT PAGET'S DISEASE

The chapter "Saving the Breast" discusses breast-saving surgeries, including central lumpectomies, which may be used to treat Paget's disease. Central lumpectomies that include the nipple and areola, and/or central quadrantectomies, often require some type of flap advancement to prevent any caving deformity of the breast after surgery. You can read more about the flap advancement procedure in "Saving the Breast."

your breast before surgery to guide the surgeon in the removal of that area. Dr. Kirsch's discussion of the use of wire localization can be found in Chapter 2, "You've Just Been Told That You Have an Abnormal Mammogram."

After the cancer has been cleared and definitive treatment (radiation and/or chemotherapy) has been rendered, the nipple and areola complex can be rebuilt by a plastic surgeon. The new nipple and areola complex should *not* be constructed at the time of your cancer surgery, because until the results from the permanent pathology report are in, it won't be known if additional treatment, such as further surgery or radiation therapy, is necessary.

CHAPTER FOUR

The Ductal Approach to Diagnosis and Treatment of Breast Cancer

By William Dooley, M.D., F.A.C.S.

For over 50 years we have known that some of the smallest and earliest breast cancers can be detected by bloody nipple discharge. Unfortunately, less than 2 percent of all breast cancers are accompanied by bloody nipple discharge. In the late 1950s, investigators tried to develop breast cancer screening based on nipple secretions. The technique of breast massage followed by nipple aspiration with a modified nursing pump, developed at the University of California, San Francisco (UCSF), was the most successful method studied. In the 1960s, UCSF researchers tested nipple aspiration fluids on over 7,000 women, showing that, although nipple aspiration detected a very small number of cancers, it identified a group of patients with atypical cells thought to be pre-malignant. These patients had a five-fold increase in breast cancer risk over ten years. This risk decreased to normal following the first ten years after the atypical cells were identified. We suspect that some pre-cancerous changes reverse while other atypical cells go on to become breast cancer. The reasons are unknown at this time, but they may have to do with dietary and environmental factors. Nonetheless, women whose breasts yielded fluid at nipple aspiration had a 1.88 relative risk of developing breast cancer, nearly twice as high as those who made no fluid.

Although these studies were elegant, little follow-up research was performed because of great skepticism in the medical community over the fate of these so-called atypical cells. In the 1980s, Dr. David Page, a breast pathologist at Vanderbilt, showed that ducts filled with atypical cells similar to those identified by nipple aspiration by the UCSF investigators were in fact precursors of ductal carcinoma in situ (DCIS) and invasive carcinoma. He also demonstrated that while not all atypical ductal hyperplasia, or ADH, lesions progressed to breast cancer, the risk for breast cancer development in women with ADH was about five times that of the usual population. This was the same incidence found in the UCSF nipple aspiration studies. Clinicians failed to have an effective treatment for these lesions and rarely identified them as a mass or a mammographic abnormality. Because of these uncertainties, breast cancer–treating physicians did not study the treatment and management of this important pre-cancerous disease in great detail.

This changed suddenly in the mid 1990s due to the success of breast cancer chemoprevention. The National Surgical Breast and Bowel Project (NSABP) performed a major study of tamoxifen versus placebo in patients at elevated risk for breast cancer to see if tamoxifen would reduce the incidence of new breast cancers. Overall, tamoxifen reduced the incidence of breast cancer by 49 percent in this study. But tamoxifen reduced the incidence of breast cancer by 80 percent in the group of patients with a history of ADH as Dr. Page described it. Now there was a reason for breast cancer–treating physicians to care about screening for ADH, because early identification of this lesion could lead to a treatment that might prevent breast cancer in the vast majority of patients.

Our major screening methods, clinical breast exam and mammography, detect ADH only rarely. By the time most physicians feel a breast cancer, it has been an invasive cancer for seven to ten years, and by the time a breast cancer is detected as a five- to six-millimeter mass on a mammogram, it has been an invasive cancer for five to seven years. Finding ADH means finding a lesion ten to twenty years before our current methods of detection. But finding ADH requires a radically new and different method of detection.

Recently several investigators joined efforts to develop a new method to screen breast secretions for ADH. Their new idea is in fact the rebirth of an old idea—washing the breast ducts for a cytology sample. This new technique was tested in a clinical trial that took place at 19 medical centers across the United States and Western Europe, and the results were published in the *Journal of The National Cancer Institute* in November 2001. Women who had a normal mammogram and physical exam but who had breasts at high risk for breast cancer were enrolled in the clinical trial. Most of the women (85 percent) produced fluid from at least one duct per breast. When lavaged, or washed with saline, these ducts produced atypical cells 24 percent of the time. In a few cases, these changes were so suspicious for cancer that, using a variety of ductal-based approaches, researchers looked for and found occult (hidden) breast cancers, most of which were early DCIS lesions. In other cases, no lesion could be found on the first attempt to lavage ducts but when the same ducts were relavaged, cancer or near-cancer cells were found.

This prompted me and a few other research physicians to attempt breast ductoscopy, which was pioneered in the early 1990s in Japan. Because the first endoscopes were large (over one millimeter in size), it was difficult to advance the scope into the ducts more than the first few centimeters. With newer multi-fiber, sub-millimeter American scopes, better images were possible, and most of the breast could be endoscoped to find a lesion. Soon after trying these new scopes it became apparent that the majority of lesions that produce atypical cells could be readily identified. Further, in women who had a known cancer, the cancer and the associated, pre-cancerous mammographically undetected lesion could be seen. We know that most women who have a recurrence in the breast after breast conservation have it in the same region as the original cancer. Now it seems obvious that this was because we did not remove the whole cancer and pre-cancerous changes the first time surgery was performed. Normally we depend on pathologists to tell us when the margins are clear of tumor and pre-cancerous changes. But endoscopy shows us that the true extent of disease is much greater than pathologists are able to detect in 55 percent of patients undergoing breast-conservation surgery.

We are at the dawn of a new age of ductal-based screening and diagnosis. Over the next several years, current methods of ductal lavage and endoscopy will become refined and joined with newer molecular screening methods. In less than 20 years, we will most likely routinely screen and treat breast cancer not as true cancer, but when it is still pre-cancerous, decades before a cancer starts. We will move from fighting a life-threatening cancer to preventing cancer before it can threaten life. Much research is needed to help us make this transition, but motivated breast cancer survivors and their female relatives who are participating in clinical trials will bring us into this new era sooner.

CHAPTER FIVE

Are You at Risk for Late Diagnosis?

By Gregory Senofsky, M.D., F.A.C.S., F.S.S.O.

There are four groups of women at risk for missed or delayed diagnosis of breast cancer: women with severe fibrocystic conditions, women with breast implants, pregnant women, and women who are breast-feeding.

• These conditions change the consistency of the normal breast and can impede physical and radiographic examination, making diagnosis of breast cancer more difficult.

• An additional problem can occur with physicians' occasional inclination to attribute a change in a woman's breast to one of these conditions rather than to a breast cancer, thus delaying consideration of biopsy, particularly in a younger woman.

• Surgeons may be less likely to biopsy women with implants, women who are pregnant, or women who are breast-feeding because of the increased risk of complications resulting from biopsy itself, although these considerations may be subliminally magnified on the surgeon's part.

If You Have Fibrocystic Breasts

Fibrocystic breasts are often painful and lumpy, which may change with your menstrual cycle and time of life. As mentioned in Chapter 1, "You've Just Discovered a Breast Lump," a fibrocystic breast condition can interfere with a mammogram, creating a dense breast that appears white on the mammogram and decreasing the visibility of a breast cancer, which also appears as white. Dense fibrocystic tissue can impede breast cancer detection by ultrasound as well. MRI (magnetic resonance imaging) is being considered as a diagnostic tool for women with severe fibrocystic disease, but it can complicate the situation and its use is still somewhat controversial. If you have fibrocystic breasts and feel a change in your breast, meticulous examination by a breast specialist is imperative. I use fine needle aspiration liberally to assess breast changes in these circumstances. When fine needle aspiration yields an atypical or suspicious result, the next step should be core needle biopsy or surgical excision. (The chapters "Saving the Breast" and "Removing Lymph Nodes" discuss breast-saving surgical options and sentinel node biopsy in detail.)

Exceptional surgical skills and judgment must be exercised in operating on women with breast cancer and severe fibrocystic breast conditions. Breast-saving surgery can often be performed, but can be technically challenging due to the firm consistency of the breast and sometimes limited mammographic assistance. It's important for everyone to consider how difficult and accurate follow-up will be after radiation therapy in the years to come. Open discussion with expert physicians providing follow-up care and excellent margins of clearance will contribute to a good long-term result. In the most severe cases of fibrocystic conditions and breast cancer, some form of mastectomy with immediate reconstruction may be required.

Cosmetic Breast Implants Make Breast Cancer Diagnosis Difficult

Women who get cosmetic breast implants rarely think about the long-term implications of their implants for future diagnosis of breast cancer.

In my lectures to women's groups, I always discuss this, because it's so important. If you have a strong family history of breast cancer and/or severe fibrocystic breasts, you should be especially cautious before choosing to undergo cosmetic breast augmentation. Once implanted, the breast is pushed forward and compressed, even with saline implants placed behind the pectoralis muscle, thus altering the breast's consistency and mammographic appearance. Often some degree of capsular contracture (tightening of the breast tissue around the implant) ensues, making physical examination and mammography even more difficult. (For more information on capsular contracture, see Chapter 9, "State-of-the-Art Breast Reconstruction.")

Biopsy of a lump or to investigate mammographic change must be performed with the utmost care in order to avoid injury to the breast implants. Mammographic abnormalities can be safely biopsied by core needle with stereotactic technology in the hands of an experienced mammographer as long as the implant can be definitively pushed out of the biopsy field. Mammographers can also safely perform ultrasound-guided aspiration or core needle biopsy if the area in question isn't too close to the implant, as the implant can be seen clearly by ultrasound. I do *not* perform needle aspiration or core needle biopsy on women with implants based on palpation (feel) alone because of the risk of injury to the implant.

If you have breast implants and a new, suspicious lump that does *not* appear on a mammogram or ultrasound, the lump should be cosmetically removed and examined by the pathologist. You and your doctor may talk about breast-saving surgery and sentinel node mapping prior to the excision (removal of the lump), because of the possibility that the lump could be found to be malignant at the time of surgery. Breast surgery on women with implants should be performed with an electrocautery instrument called a Bovie, using the dull Bovie tip so as to prevent cutting or ripping the implant. (Electrocautery uses an electric current to cut or coagulate.) Sharp instruments should be avoided. If the implant is old, mammography

IF YOU HAVE BREAST IMPLANTS AND NOTICE A CHANGE IN YOUR BREAST

Consider seeking the second opinion of a breast surgeon after talking to your plastic surgeon. The change may not be due to the implant.

or MRI can be performed preoperatively to show that the implant is intact prior to the biopsy or surgery.

Radiation can induce significant capsular contracture, sometimes requiring removal of the implant (capsulectomy or capsulotomy) and implant replacement. Occasionally the final cosmetic result of breast-saving surgery and radiation therapy will be unacceptable to a woman with implants, and skin-sparing mastectomy with a TRAM flap may become necessary. (To learn more about TRAM flap, see Chapter 9, "State-of-the-Art Breast Reconstruction.")

If you have breast implants and you notice a change in your breasts, think twice before accepting a diagnosis that the change is due to the implant without first having a biopsy. I've seen some real tragedies in which women with implants developed a lump or skin change in their breast and were told by a doctor that the lump or change was due to the implant and thus no biopsy was recommended. If you visit a plastic surgeon with complaints about a lump or change in your breast, and the plastic surgeon feels that the lump or change is due to the implant, a second opinion by a breast cancer surgeon may be in order. Biopsy, when performed correctly, will provide the answer and will not tear the implant. Breast skin erythema, or redness, in a woman with or without implants should never be assumed to be cellulitis (a skin infection). Inflammatory breast cancer, a rare aggressive form of breast cancer, which appears as thick, reddened breast skin, must also be considered and ruled out by skin biopsy, if the redness does not resolve quickly with antibiotics and the ultrasound shows no underlying abscess. This is a simple procedure in which a tiny piece of skin is taken and sent to the pathologist for analysis. It can be done under local anesthetic with a few tiny sutures.

Some challenging decision-making occurs when a woman already treated with mastectomy and implant reconstruction (possibly with radiation therapy) develops a new change in the reconstructed breast. These situations almost always require careful biopsy by a breast surgeon to rule out recurrent breast cancer.

Pregnancy and Breast Cancer

Pregnancy not only makes diagnosis of breast cancer more difficult, it can exacerbate breast cancer when it does occur. Pregnancy can cause significant changes in both the size and shape of the breast and can promote the growth of benign tumors, such as fibroadenomas. But it can also cause malignant tumors to increase in size rapidly because of the increase in estrogen in the body. Pregnancy can cause breast skin to swell, creating a thick red texture. Pregnancy can also propel an inflammatory breast cancer, which also appears as thickened, reddened skin. In these situations, skin biopsy is often indicated to rule out inflammatory breast cancer, unless it clears rapidly with antibiotics. Due to the risk to the fetus, pregnant women cannot have mammograms; however, ultrasound is very safe and can be extremely helpful to assess a cyst versus a solid mass. Solid masses or complex cysts that are not particularly suspicious should be biopsied immediately with fine needle aspiration or core needle biopsy. If there is any significant level of suspicion, a needle biopsy followed by a wide excisional biopsy should be performed with additional sentinel node mapping, if the tumor is cancerous. Sentinel node mapping in pregnancy is considered safe. There is no evidence to indicate that the radioactive tracer is harmful to a fetus because the dose is so small as to be considered insignificant and without risk. The blue dye method of sentinel node mapping has also shown no evidence of adverse reactions in pregnancy; however, there have been rare cases of allergic reactions to the blue dye.

Because mammography, radiation therapy, and chemotherapy are not compatible with a living fetus, the overall treatment of breast cancer in pregnant women is complex. The timing of diagnosis in relation to the trimester of pregnancy is important. Breast cancer found in the third trimester can often be treated with breast-saving surgery immediately, while radiation and/or chemotherapy are delayed until the child is born. Breast cancer diagnosed in the first or second trimester may be treated with mastectomy. In this situation, I would recommend a delayed reconstruction. Very aggressive breast cancer found in the first or second trimester forces an extremely difficult discussion regarding the risk of carrying the pregnancy to term. This discussion should involve the patient and all of her treating physicians, including the OB/GYN.

I cannot overemphasize the importance of an accurate biopsy to diagnose a perceived abnormality in the breast of a pregnant woman. Needle biopsies and superficial biopsies can be easily performed under local anesthesia. The physician or nurse practitioner who thinks that he or she is doing a pregnant patient an "emotional favor" by reassuring her and avoiding biopsy may in fact be risking the life of both mother and child.

Lactation, or the production of breast milk, often makes diagnosis of a breast lump or other change in the breast difficult. Although most lumps that appear during lactation are benign, including lactating adenomas (solid benign tumors) or milk cysts (trapped collections of milk), breast cancer can also appear during the lactation period. Surgeons and radiologists are typically leery of performing biopsy in a lactating breast because of the risk of creating a milk fistula, or milk leakage, through the incision. Milk fistulas can complicate the wound and possibly become infected.

If you are breast-feeding and notice a new lump in your breast, see a breast surgeon and have a breast ultrasound. Mammography is not helpful in the lactating breast. I have performed fine needle aspiration many times in lactating breasts

> **IF YOU ARE BREAST-FEEDING AND SCHEDULED FOR BREAST SURGERY**
>
> I recommend stopping breast-feeding immediately and undergoing a two- to three-week period of firm breast binding to decrease the risk of milk fistula. Breast binding can be done with a bias wrap (a thin cotton cloth or ACE wrap that you can obtain through your gynecologist, a medical supply store, or high-quality pharmacy) around the chest and breast area, rewrapping at least once a day. No medications are necessary to stop lactation. Following this two- to three-week period, breast surgery can be performed with excellent results.

and have never seen a milk fistula develop. Fine needle aspiration may resolve a milk cyst or suggest the diagnosis of a solid tumor. Should fine needle aspiration be suspicious or atypical, core needle biopsy can then be performed. The risk of milk fistula following core needle biopsy is extraordinarily low, especially if only one or two cores are obtained with a number 18-gauge core needle biopsy gun.

Women who are breast-feeding are prone to mastitis (an infection similar to cellulitis), breast abscess, and nipple trauma. Initially an OB/GYN or lactation specialist can treat these conditions. A woman with a breast abscess will often be referred to a surgeon. A breast abscess is a collection of pus in the breast that requires removal of the pus and antibiotic treatment. Breast abscesses appear spontaneously or sometimes develop during breast-feeding. In general, I do not operate on breast abcesses, but rather drain out all the pus with a needle in the office and place the woman on antibiotics. If the abscess continues to reform, the aspiration process can be done again. Typically, breast-feeding can be continued. In rare instances, surgery is required; a small plastic drain may have to be placed via a tiny incision to continuously evacuate the abscess, thus allowing it to heal. Larger incisions with abscess cavity packing (daily changing of a sterilize cloth ribbon packed into the cavity) can ultimately be deforming and is usually unnecessary for the vast majority of breast abscesses. As I mentioned previously, quick skin biopsy is required when a woman has a persistently reddened breast that does not clear up with antibiotics.

CHAPTER SIX

Saving the Breast

By Gregory Senofsky, M.D., F.A.C.S., F.S.S.O.

It's been almost three months since I had my surgery. I can't tell a difference in the size of my breast. I have sensation everywhere except on a spot by the side of my incision. I'm pleased with the way my breast looks. It looks almost better than before surgery. • Cynthia

I went down an entire bra size, but if you look at me, the breast that had cancer still looks like a breast, and I have total sensation, which was important to me. I have a very slight scar. It looks completely natural. I am thrilled with the cosmetic outcome of my breast cancer surgery. If the way your breast looks is important to you, I would not go to a general surgeon but seek out someone who does this surgery all of the time.
• Anne

You can barely see my incision line, and I had two tumors taken out (in the same quadrant). I would be very surprised if anyone could tell me where my scar is in another year and a half. It's just the finest little line.
• Beverly

I was really fortunate that my surgeon was able to remove the cancer and give me a good-looking breast, which looks better than the other one.
• Joan

> *I think many women go into surgery thinking that that they will be disfigured. But there are doctors out there who really care what a woman looks like after surgery. I'm happy with the appearance of my breast and my scar. I call it my beautiful scar.* • Linda R.

> *My breast is smaller than the other one, but I was shocked that it looked so good. It looks better than the other one.* • Francine

Most small- to mid-sized breast cancers can be treated with breast-conserving surgeries—that is surgeries that remove part, rather than all, of the breast tissue, often in addition to radiation treatment. Although surgeons have been using breast-saving procedures since the 1970s, much has changed in the field since then. Until recently, women with breast cancer were given the single option of modified radical mastectomy or lumpectomy (for small breast cancers) with axillary node dissection (the complete removal of lymph nodes to detect the spread of cancer) and radiation treatment. Today there are additional choices, including larger tailored lumpectomies or quadrantectomies with flap advancement closures, which involves the removal of up to a quarter of the breast tissue and immediate reconstruction using a woman's own

BREAST-SAVING SURGERY FOR BREAST CANCER WITH POSITIVE COSMETIC RESULTS

I view breast-saving surgery for breast cancer differently than I did when I finished my training as a surgeon. I now understand that better techniques allow surgeons to do larger lumpectomies and quadrantectomies, get widely clear margins, reduce the risk of local recurrence, and sometimes even improve the shape of the breast. These techniques require an artistic approach and can be thought of as targeted internal sculpting.

Surgeons are always concerned about making the breast look worse after large lumpectomies. Few surgeons understand that with the proper use of flap advancement, volume redistribution, and mastopexy (breast lift), one can sometimes make the breast look better, even if it will be smaller, depending on the location of the cancer in the breast. This may require the services of a plastic surgeon to reshape the opposite breast to match the breast that has undergone surgery, but many patients are extremely happy with the look of their new breasts.

breast tissue. Additional surgical options for reconstructing very large lumpectomy defects include a procedure called a latissimus dorsi flap, which I discuss later in this chapter. Preoperative bracketing localization wire placement guided by mammography or ultrasound to help the surgeon locate a breast cancer's outer edges when it can't be felt is another recent improvement as is sentinel node mapping, which may be more accurate and less invasive than axillary node dissection.

For more about sentinel node biopsy and axillary node dissection, see Chapter 8, "Removing Lymph Nodes.") In this chapter, we will take a look at some newer options for breast-saving surgery. You'll find an in-depth discussion of radiation treatment in Chapter 11, "Radiotherapy: What to Know, What to Ask."

These newer surgical techniques for breast-conserving surgery have the advantage of allowing an experienced surgeon to completely remove a larger or nonpalpable breast cancer along with a significant rim of healthy breast tissue around it (called the *margin of clearance*) to greatly reduce the chance that cancer will recur in the breast and at the same time to reconstruct the breast with a woman's own breast tissue so that her breast often looks the same, and sometimes even better, than before surgery. The national rate for local recurrence (cancer coming back near the lumpectomy site) is approximately 7 to 12 percent. My current isolated local recurrence rate using these newer techniques is currently running noticeably lower than most reported studies. Dr. Umberto Veronesi of Italy, perhaps the most renowned breast surgeon in the world, has a local recurrence rate following quadrantectomy of 2.6 percent. I am convinced that these improved local recurrence rates are due to wider margins of clearance at the time of surgery.

| HMO SURVIVAL TIPS

If you are told you need a mastectomy, strongly consider getting a second opinion with a breast surgeon, even if your HMO won't pay for it. Also consider meeting with a plastic surgeon for consideration of immediate breast reconstruction, if mastectomy is truly needed.

Does your HMO have a breast surgeon? If your HMO doesn't have a breast surgeon, call your HMO to find out whether you have a point-of-service plan (POS), in which you can choose a doctor outside of the plan.

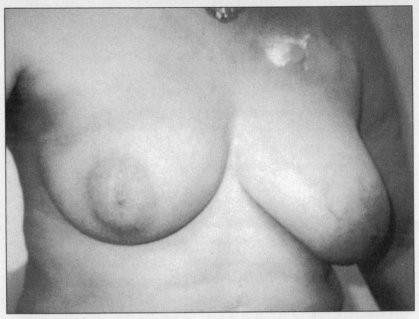

Figure 2. Improved Cosmetic Result after Large Lumpectomy with Flap Advancement Closure.

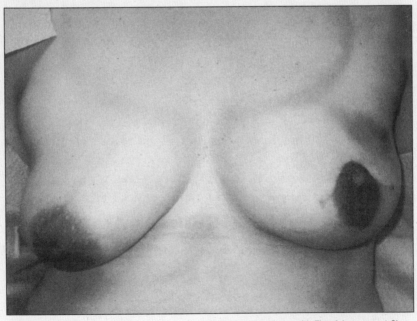

Figure 3. Improved Cosmetic Result after Large Central Lumpectomy with Flap Advancement Closure. This patient will undergo cosmetic surgery of her other breast to match the breast with the lumpectomy.

Are You a Candidate for Breast-Conserving Surgery?

If you can have all of your cancer removed with a clear margin (we'll talk about this concept shortly) and still be satisfied with the appearance of your breast postoperatively, you're a good candidate for breast-saving surgery, as long as you can receive postoperative radiation therapy to your breast, if necessary. The size of your tumor, which is determined not just by touch, but also by mammogram and ultrasound, will be a very important factor in making this decision. Secondly, the size of your tumor in relation to the size of your breast must be considered. For example, a woman with small breasts who has a very large tumor or extensive DCIS (ductal carcinoma in situ, a type of cancer that is confined to the milk ducts, but which can be widespread in the breast) may be a better candidate for mastectomy. The exact location of the tumor in the breast is of paramount concern. A very large tumor in the middle of the breast or the lower part of the breast, for example, may also be better treated with a mastectomy and immediate reconstruction.

Breast-conserving therapy can sometimes change the shape and size of your breast. If you have a large tumor, your affected breast may be smaller than the other postoperatively (what is critical is the *shape* of your postoperative breast), although additional surgery can be done to match or reduce your opposite breast. This is one of the reasons why it's important to think about the possible need for breast reconstruction, even if you're planning to have breast-conserving therapy, and to talk at length with your breast surgeon about all of your options so that you'll know what the results of surgery are likely to be. In the right hands, breast-conserving surgery can sometimes improve the shape of your breast.

Sometimes chemotherapy can be used to shrink a very large tumor before surgery. This might be considered when a tumor measures more than four centimeters in diameter or in a situation that could potentially convert a woman who is a candidate for mastectomy into a candidate for breast-saving surgery, although this is still somewhat controversial and highly individualized. It does not appear that preoperative chemotherapy significantly improves overall survival results and there is a risk that the cancer may not be responsive to the chemotherapy and continue to grow during treatment.

Women who cannot tolerate or adamantly reject radiation may also be better candidates for mastectomy, although radiation may sometimes be necessary even after mastectomy. Here again, you'll want to ask your breast surgeon how radiation treatment will affect your choice of breast-conserving therapy over mastectomy. You should also be aware that radiation treatment could change the size and shape of your breast.

A margin of clearance is the least amount of normal tissue between the edge of the breast cancer and the edge of the lumpectomy and is measured in millimeters. Studies have shown that removing all of the cancer with a clear rim of normal tissue (in which no cancer cells are present) is critical to controlling recurrence of cancer in the breast. In other words, when we can get all the cancer out, the chance of cancer coming back in your breast in the future is significantly reduced. A more difficult situation arises, however, if cancer has spread to other areas outside of the breast at the time of detection. While it's always critical to get all of the cancer out to try to avoid a recurrence of cancer in the breast, additional systemic treatments, such as chemotherapy or hormone therapy, take on a more prominent role in treatment when cancer has already spread.

Currently there are no standards for an acceptable margin of clearance except simply to say that cancer should not be present at the margins of the lumpectomy. Clinical research is ongoing in this area, but studies are now available that demonstrate lower rates of local recurrence when good margins of clearance are obtained at surgery. I advocate a five- to ten-millimeter microscopic margin of clearance when I do lumpectomies and will generally accept no less than a five-millimeter margin, unless there are extenuating circumstances.[1] To try to make sure I get good margins, I perform surgery with a pathologist present in the operating room. Once the tumor is out, the pathologist can then immediately measure the margin of clearance, and margins that appear too close can then be re-excised (removed) right away under the pathologist's direction. Final pathology results are typically available one to two

---

[1] Some surgeons will accept as little as a one-millimeter margin of clearance, but I strongly disagree with this.

WHAT TYPE OF SURGERY ARE YOU HAVING? DEFINITIONS.

The terms for breast cancer surgeries can be very confusing. Although it's vital to ask your doctor to describe in detail the surgery you are having, here is a list of terms and definitions that can aid in your discussions.

Excisional biopsy: simple removal of a small lump or nodule with no attention to microscopic margins.

Lumpectomy (also called wide excision): removal of a lump or radiographic tumor with a simultaneous attempt to clear the margins of suspected or documented breast cancer. In my practice, I utilize flap advancement when nooooooary to prevent a dimpling deformity.

Cosmetic quadrantectomy: removal of approximately 25 percent of the breast with an attempt to clear the margins of a larger breast cancer. This is done with a flap advancement in my practice.

Central quadrantectomy: a quadrantectomy that includes the nipple and areola.

Simple mastectomy: removal of the breast without removal of the lymph nodes.

Modified radical mastectomy: removal of the breast with appropriate lymph nodes under the arm.

Skin-sparing mastectomy: removal of the breast with a minimal amount of skin necessary to effectively clear the margins. This is performed in concert with immediate reconstruction.

days later and sometimes will indicate the need for further surgery. When I re-excise edges of a lumpectomy cavity, I generally remove one centimeter of tissue width with the *prior* pathology report in the operating room so that I know exactly which area to remove. I strongly recommend discussing the intended margin of clearance in millimeters with your surgeon *prior* to surgery. If a close margin (less than two millimeters) is acceptable to your surgeon, consider a second opinion. If you have DCIS, I *strongly* recommend at least a five-millimeter margin of clearance to

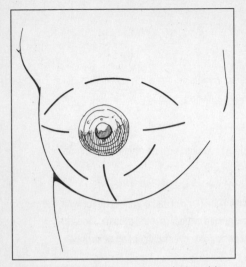

Figure 3A. Orientation for lumpectomy/wide excision.

minimize the risk of recurrence. Insist on knowing the final margins of clearance on the pathology report after surgery (the permanent pathology report) and discuss this with all of your doctors. In addition to discussing the intended margin size with your surgeon prior to lumpectomy, ask your surgeon what his or her local recurrence rates are. Again, if your surgeon cannot give you an answer, consider getting a second opinion.

In a small percentage of individuals, mastectomy may ultimately be required, if the cancer extends far out microscopically in the breast away from the palpable lump or mammographic appearance of the tumor. This type of "silent" extension is unusual, but when it occurs, only the pathologist can detect it.

What Does Breast-Conserving Surgery Involve?

It's likely that you'll hear a variety of terms to describe removal of cancer in the breast with *lumpectomy* or *wide excision* being the most common. You may also hear the term *partial mastectomy*. I use the terms *lumpectomy* and *wide excision* interchangeably, although lumpectomy is a kind of misnomer as it can also be used to refer to the removal of any significant breast lump as well as cancers that can't be felt. Lumpectomy (also called *wide excision*) is an outpatient surgical procedure in which a breast mass is removed with a rim of normal breast tissue left attached to it in all directions. We can do this operation at the time of excisional biopsy, but I prefer a preoperative needle aspiration or biopsy in most cases. I cannot stress how vital it is to understand that until the final pathology results are in, we will not know whether we have gotten clear margins or not. In cases where clear margins are not obtained, additional surgery will be necessary to get clear margins. Several studies now show that clear margins after lumpectomy are critical to minimizing the risk of cancer coming back in the breast in the region of the original tumor.

Newer Artistic Techniques Provide Better Cosmetic Results With Large Lumpectomies

When a lump or mass is removed from the breast, a cavity often remains. Small cavities fill with fluid and retain their shape, but larger cavities often cave in, especially after radiation therapy.

In my practice, when the cavity is significant, I often reconstruct it using a woman's own breast tissue in a procedure known as *flap advancement.* Flap advancement redistributes the remaining breast tissue and helps minimize the caving or dimpling deformity after lumpectomy. This can be done immediately after lumpectomy or quadrantectomy when the pathologist has completed his initial evaluation of the specimen and while you are still under anesthesia. In this procedure, the back edges of the breast radiating away from the cavity are gently separated from the tissue in front of the chest wall muscle and then brought together in a way that shapes the breast well. Flap advancement does

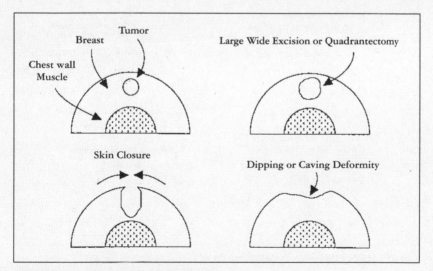

Figure 4. Large Wide Excision or Quadrantectomy.

not disorient the remaining cavity edges in the event that additional removal of a portion or all of the cavity wall is required. The skin is then closed with cosmetic precision. To help you visualize the nature of the operation and the results, take a look at the diagram below. Large lumpectomies and flap advancements when performed correctly can tighten the breast and sometimes lift it, yielding excellent cosmetic results.

The judicious removal of an ellipse of skin directly over the lumpectomy defect is another important technical maneuver done to avoid dipping or caving in the breast after a lumpectomy. The subcutaneous fat can be reduced into the cavity and the skin edges can be cosmetically closed. When combined with flap advancement, this maneuver greatly limits dipping and promotes an excellent, firm, and even surface. If the cancer is close to the skin, an ellipse of skin will definitely have to be taken to get a good margin of clearance.

If you have small- to mid-sized breasts and have had a very large lumpectomy or quadrantectomy, a latissimus dorsi flap can be performed. This procedure involves the use of skin and muscle from your back to reconstruct the lumpectomy site and can be done when flap advancement alone will not provide a good enough cosmetic result. It's

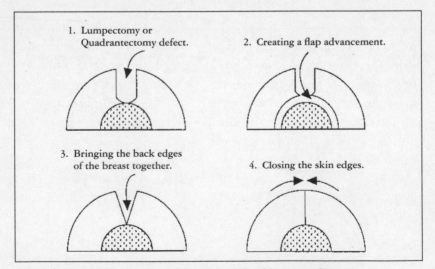

Figure 5. Large Wide Excision or Quadrantectomy with Flap Advancement Closure

a much more extensive operation, involving more time and recovery than a flap advancement, so you'll want to talk to your breast surgeon and plastic surgeon about this procedure in detail, if you desire it or if it's suggested to you. (Also see the Chapter 9, "State-of-the-Art Breast Reconstruction.")

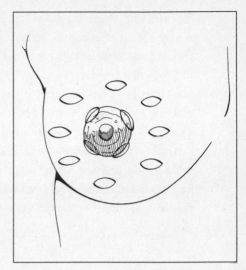

Figure 5A. Orientation for elliptical incisions.

Sometimes a breast lift (mastopexy) can be done as part of high-quality post-lumpectomy reconstruction for breast cancers in the upper central or upper outer quadrants of the breast. When the lifted breast is significantly improved, the other breast can be lifted to match. But I suggest waiting to do this until all of your treatment is done, including radiation therapy to the breast.

A small implant should never be used as part of the reconstruction of a larger lumpectomy defect. This has been tried and has consistently failed due to the rejection of the small implant within the breast tissue.

Cosmetic quadrantectomy[2] is a new technique that is used when lumpectomy would fail or has already failed to obtain clear microscopic margins. This is essentially a larger lumpectomy, or wider excision, with larger flap advancement and can be used to treat cancers from one to one-and-a-half inches in diameter and, in some cases, even cancers up to two inches in diameter, depending on the size of your breast.

Developed by Umberto Veronesi, quadrantectomy, or removal of a quarter or more of the breast tissue in a segmental distribution, produces better local control than regular lumpectomies in situations in which wide margins can't be obtained with standard lumpectomy. The quadrantectomy adaptation that combines the procedure with flap advancement

---

[2] G.M. Senofsky, E.D. Gierson, P.H. Craig, P.P. Gamagami, M.J. Silverstein, "Local Excision, Lumpectomy, and Quadrantectomy: Surgical Considerations," *Surgery of the Breast: Principles and Art,* edited by Scott L. Spear. Lippincott-Raven Publishers: Philadelphia, 1998.

for excellent cosmetic results was developed at the Van Nuys Breast Center by a team of breast surgeons and plastic surgeons. Cosmetic quadrantectomy has tremendous potential for helping women with breast cancer to keep their breasts.

Many surgeons feel that if the nipple and areola (the dark skin surrounding your nipple) must be removed, the breast can't be conserved. I strongly disagree and routinely perform large central lumpectomy and central quadrantectomy with flap advancement, obtaining excellent cosmetic results and wide margins of clearance. Generally the nipple and a portion of the areola can be taken with a nice cosmetic result still possible. A nipple and areola can always be reconstructed at a later time by a plastic surgeon, if the entire area must be removed. It is unlikely that you will have feeling in a reconstructed nipple, although occasionally some women do have feeling in this area when the areola is spared. The breast size is slightly reduced after central quadrantectomy, seen most notably in profile.

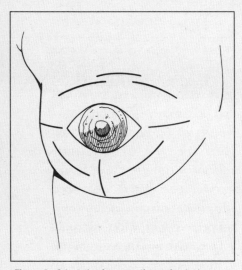

Figure 6. Orientation for cosmetic quadrantectomy incisions.

The way in which your surgeon makes the incision for breast surgery makes a tremendous difference in the cosmetic outcome. In general, incisions should be in the direction of the natural skin lines in the breast or periareolar area (around your areola). Vertical incisions should not be used except occasionally for lower breast lesions requiring larger lumpectomies or quadrantectomies and flap advancements. No incision should be made without considering how it will affect mastectomy should it be necessary later on.

Some breast cancers, such as DCIS, small cancers, or deep cancers cannot be felt in the breast. Here, it's critical to place one or more sterile wires into the breast at the site of the cancer before surgery to increase the chances of getting a clear margin at surgery. This is done by the radiologist preoperatively and is called *wire localization*. In many practices, only one wire is used, but the relatively new practice of using more than one wire placed around the edges of the tumor can improve the likelihood of getting all of the cancer out with a clear margin. In fact, the high incidence of positive margins after surgery using a single hooked wire led to the development of the technique of bracketing a lesion that can't be felt. Using local anesthesia, an experienced mammographer will place localization wires into your breast around the tumor in the radiology suite before surgery using mammography or ultrasound to visualize the cancer. Dr. Kirsch discusses this further in Chapter 2, "You've Just Been Told That You Have an Abnormal Mammogram."

I typically perform sentinel lymph node mapping at the same time as breast cancer surgery. The lymph nodes are small glands that are part of your immune system and help protect you from bacteria, viruses, and other microorganisms. The lymph nodes under the armpit are often the first place to which breast cancer spreads. We remove the nodes most likely to contain cancer to see if it has spread and to make further treatment decisions, if it has. When a breast pathologist is present in the operating room, he or she can give an immediate impression of the sentinel node or nodes. (For more information about removing lymph nodes, see Chapter 8, "Removing Lymph Nodes.")

If you have breast implants and require breast surgery, there are special considerations to discuss with your doctor. I use similar techniques for lumpectomy and flap advancement closure for women with implants, but common sense dictates that no needles or sharp instruments should be used near the implant. To prevent implant rupture, I do these operations with a dull electrocautery and dull instruments. Clearly you will want to make sure that your implant is intact and not disrupted prior to any surgery. Sometimes a woman with implants will be unaware that her implant is leaking. Mammography and sometimes MRI can be used to detect silicone leakage, while a leaking saline implant will be deflated. You should know, too, that radiation treatment to a breast with an implant could induce a phenomenon called *capsular contracture*, a tightening of the breast tissue around the implant that can cause pain and a tight breast that appears contracted. (See Chapter 5, "Are You at Risk for Late Diagnosis?")

Pregnancy is another special circumstance that requires a high degree of individualized care and collaboration between a woman's gynecologist, breast surgeon, and radiologist, who must all have close and frequent discussions about any abnormal findings on a pregnant woman's physical examination or ultrasound. As I mentioned previously, a woman who discovers an abnormality in her breast while pregnant must get a diagnosis immediately because the increased levels of estrogen present during pregnancy can sometimes stimulate breast cancer growth. Conservative breast cancer surgery can generally be performed during the later phases of pregnancy, although radiation should be avoided until after delivery because of the risk to the baby.

Rarely a palpable lymph node in the axilla will be biopsied and determined to be from a breast cancer, although no signs of breast cancer are present on examination or mammogram. Ultrasound and/or MRI will sometimes be of assistance and every attempt at image guided needle biopsy should be explored if any lesion can be seen in the breast by an experienced radiologist. If, after appropriate testing, the medical oncologist finds no other signs of spread, a decision must be made as to the treatment of the breast and axilla. I usually recommend an axillary node dissection and a large lumpectomy or quadrantectomy focusing on the upper outer quadrant of the breast where the majority of breast cancer occurs. This can then be followed by radiation and chemotherapy. No surgery to the breast but radiation therapy to the breast is another option, and some patients will desire a mastectomy although the therapeutic advantage of mastectomy in this situation is unproven. Chemotherapy is usually given.

Who Can Perform Breast-Conserving Surgery?

Although breast-conserving surgery has been in use for decades, there are still few standards for these procedures, and the results can vary widely as they are quite "operator-dependent," requiring both skilled targeting of the cancer and an artistic approach. It's relatively easy for an inexperienced surgeon to remove a tiny breast cancer with a clear margin and achieve a good cosmetic result. But the real surgical finesse comes into play when a woman has a larger tumor in a smaller breast, for example cup size B or smaller. An experienced breast surgeon can perform these surgeries while a surgeon with less experience may provide you with less than optimal results or resort to performing a mastectomy. Many surgeons, even some breast surgeons, may not be fully trained to do large lumpectomies or quadrantectomies with truly excellent cosmetic results.

If lumpectomy is offered to you to treat a mid- to large-sized breast cancer, ask what techniques will be employed to reconstruct any defect in your breast caused by your surgery. If no reconstructive technique is offered, you might want to find a surgeon who can offer this advantage.

I can't emphasize how important it is to understand the nature of any options you are given for breast cancer surgery and how much the outcome can depend on your surgeon's experience. Many of the techniques discussed here, including reconstructing lumpectomy defects and reshaping a woman's breast with her own breast tissue after larger lumpectomies while maintaining widely clear margins, are unfamiliar concepts to some surgeons. Your health matters. The appearance of your breast after surgery matters. Be good to yourself. Ask questions. Learn about the most sophisticated options that are available to you. Find out about your surgeon's qualifications to do breast cancer surgery. Consider a second opinion. Although your initial response to a cancer diagnosis may be to have the cancer removed as soon as possible, you do have time to make treatment decisions. Never hesitate to demand the best and latest in treatment and care.

CHAPTER SEVEN

Will You Need a Mastectomy?

By Gregory Senofsky, M.D., F.A.C.S., F.S.S.O.

Having a mastectomy didn't make me feel less of a woman than before. I'll say I'm different but better in every way. I'm very proud of myself. When I went back to work, I told everybody about it without having shame anymore. I was alive! And that was what mattered to me.
• Patricia

People are not the sum of their parts. Losing a breast doesn't change who you are. The experience of cancer may change you, but not losing a breast. My breast was not important to me, living was important to me.
• Joelle

It was more important to me to be healthy than to be "whole." • Linda L.

One of the most difficult issues a woman diagnosed with breast cancer will have to face is whether or not a mastectomy will be a part of her initial treatment for breast cancer. Losing a breast or breasts can be traumatic. You may or may not place tremendous importance on your breasts, but the important thing to remember is that your feelings about your breasts and the potential loss of a breast or breasts are to be respected and fully considered as you and your doctor make decisions about surgery. This is your time, your health, and your body. You should never be rushed or pressured into a decision about surgery until you have all the facts about your diagnosis and your treatment plan. Remember, your cancer is unique to you—it's unlike any other woman's—and what is right for other women will not necessarily be right for you.

Mastectomy has undergone a significant evolution since the turn of the twentieth century when Dr. William Stuart Halsted first developed it at Johns Hopkins University in Baltimore. At the time, breast cancer was always diagnosed late when there was extensive breast and axillary involvement (involvement of the lymph nodes in the armpit region) and, often, involvement of the major chest wall muscle. The operation, which took the breast, the lymph nodes under the arm, and both major and minor chest wall muscles, was mutilating and debilitating, but it was the only operation available at the time that worked.

In the 1950s and 1960s, the modified radical mastectomy was introduced, sparing women with breast cancer the removal of the major chest wall muscle (pectoralis major), and in most cases, the pectoralis minor. The results were equal to those of the radical mastectomy. When mammography became available, it was possible to detect breast cancer at a significantly earlier stage in its progress, and in the 1970s, Dr. George Crile introduced breast-saving surgery. (Breast-saving surgeries are discussed in Chapter 6, "Saving the Breast.") Radiation therapy in combination with high-quality breast-saving surgery has been closely examined in clinical trials, yielding equivalent survival results to modified radical mastectomy when the cancer can be well-excised (removed) with a clear margin.

How Is a Mastectomy Done?

A mastectomy is the removal of the breast gland. Before surgery, while you are under anesthesia, the surgeon will determine where to make the incision for the mastectomy. He or she will begin by separating the skin and fat away from the breast, raising what is known as *skin flaps*. The breast is removed, typically through a relatively small incision, unless there is cancer near the skin or no reconstruction is planned. The chest muscles are left alone. It's very important that the surgeon know the

ASK YOUR DOCTOR HOW THE SKIN ENVELOPE WILL BE CREATED FOR YOUR MASTECTOMY

Ask your surgeon how he or she will make the skin flaps for your mastectomy, and make sure that your surgeon does not use electrocautery for this part of the surgery. Electrocautery is an electrical surgical tool. I don't approve of this technique because this can burn the skin or make the skin flaps too thick, leaving more breast tissue attached to them. There are other techniques that can be used to make skin flaps, including scissors, scalpel, or the harmonic scalpel, a relatively new surgical tool that cuts tissue with an ultrasonic vibration.

anatomy of the axilla (the underarm where the lymph nodes are situated) extremely well, because there are several nerves and blood vessels there that must be carefully treated during surgery.

Once the breast is removed, it will go to the pathology lab for evaluation to make sure the cancer has been removed, that the margins are clear, and to evaluate the lymph nodes. The margins at the edge of the cancer must be well-cleared from the skin and muscle to minimize local recurrence. The pathologist should come into the operating room to review the margins with the surgeon prior to closure.

Axillary lymph node dissection or sentinel node biopsy is usually done at the same time as mastectomy. (See Chapter 8, "Removing Lymph Nodes.") In some cases, lymph node removal may not be required, for example, if you are quite elderly or sickly with clinically negative lymph nodes, if you have predominately low-grade DCIS, or an extremely early and tiny cancer but cannot tolerate radiation therapy.

Reconstructive surgery can be an incredible advantage to those who desire it. Dr. Jensen will cover options for reconstruction in depth in Chapter 9, "State-of-the-Art Breast Reconstruction." I must say that the women in my practice who have had truly expert reconstruction immediately in conjunction with mastectomy tend to feel confident and optimistic. Important considerations include the quality of the reconstruction, how the skin flaps are created, and how much skin is removed. The surgeon performing the mastectomy should work closely with the plastic and reconstructive surgeon before surgery to plan the incision, and the plastic surgeon should strongly consider assisting the breast cancer surgeon in the operating room before reconstruction. In this way, the two surgeons can make a better judgment about how much skin to take or leave for the best cosmetic results, as well as the best oncologic results.

If mastectomy is recommended, ask your surgeon:

- How big is the tumor?

- Exactly what are the indications to do the mastectomy?

- What is your breast-saving surgery to mastectomy rate? The surgeon's breast-saving surgery rate should be 65 percent or more in communities where mammography is widely available.

- What is the largest lump you would remove in a lumpectomy in a breast of my size?

- Is there any benefit to giving chemotherapy first to shrink the cancer? (This is still fairly controversial in terms of risks and results, but it is something to discuss with your doctor.)

- How much skin would you remove in my mastectomy?

If you are interested in reconstruction, ask:

- Is there any reason not to do immediate reconstruction?

- Who is the best plastic surgeon in this area for breast reconstruction?

- Will the plastic surgeon assist you during the mastectomy or at least help you plan the incision?

The possibility of radiation therapy after surgery will affect your choice of reconstruction. If radiation therapy is planned, I do not recommend breast implants, because radiation can greatly increase the risk of a phenomenon called *capsular contracture*, a painful tightening of the breast tissue around the implant. Other reconstructive techniques that employ your own tissue to create a breast can be radiated with excellent results.

Is Mastectomy the Best Treatment for You?

Most of the women I see in my practice can be treated with breast-saving surgeries. But about 25 to 30 percent of the people I see with breast cancer will need a mastectomy. It is surprising to note that in certain areas of the country, mastectomy is still highly utilized when other options could be made available. This is due in large part to the opinions and technical ability of the treating physicians, especially the surgeons. Sometimes a surgeon will offer a woman a mastectomy simply because the surgeon can't get a good cosmetic result with a large lumpectomy. Many surgeons believe that if the nipple/areolar complex must be resected (removed), mastectomy is required, but this is not necessarily the case. If you are offered a mastectomy as the first choice of surgical treatment for breast cancer, ask the surgeon exactly what the indications are for mastectomy in your case and consider getting a second opinion.

Some Reasons Why You May Need a Mastectomy

Mastectomy may be your optimal surgical treatment for breast cancer if:

• You have a cancer that is truly too large relative to your breast size to remove with good cosmetic results or if you have a mammogram that is uninterpretable (for example, if you have severe fibrocystic breasts or extensive microcalcifications) because we won't be able to follow you postoperatively with mammography. It's necessary to follow you with mammography to watch for possible recurrences of cancer.

• If you cannot tolerate the radiation therapy that accompanies breast-saving surgery—for instance, if you have a collagen vascular disease, such as lupus or scleroderma. Likewise, if you have had radiation therapy in the past for Hodgkin's disease, you may be a better candidate for mastectomy. It's important to note that radiation in addition to mastectomy may be necessary for some women. This can happen when a tumor is close to the chest wall or when a woman has a larger cancer and a significant amount of axillary lymph node involvement.

• If you have had breast-saving surgery with radiotherapy in the past for breast cancer and you develop a new breast cancer in the radiated breast.

• If you cannot get to a facility to receive radiation treatment.

• If you have multiple breast cancers or two cancers in separate areas of the breast that cannot be removed by a single large lumpectomy or quadrantectomy.

• Women who are pregnant must avoid radiation until after delivery. Nonetheless, a woman who is pregnant may still be a candidate for breast-conserving surgery during the last trimester. Women diagnosed with breast cancer during the first or second trimester will likely require mastectomy if the cancer is invasive.

• In a minority of cases, a mastectomy may be necessary after initial breast-saving surgery if we cannot get a rim of normal breast tissue between the cancer and the edge of the lumpectomy, referred to as a *clear margin*. Occasionally some types of cancer cannot be seen on a mammogram, or portions of the cancer cannot be seen on the mammogram and the cancer is actually significantly larger than it appears mammographically. Rarely there are mammographically invisible satellites of cancer that extend millimeters away from the main cancer, significantly increasing the volume of tissue that must be removed in order to obtain a clear margin.

We got the results back from the biopsy pretty quickly. I had cancer again, which was surprising because my first cancer had been small and easily containable. I hadn't had reconstruction with the first set of surgeries because it wasn't necessary. But there wasn't enough breast left to do another partial, so I had a modified radical mastectomy. • Joelle

The Type and Extent of Your Cancer Matters

Ductal carcinoma in situ (DCIS) is a preinvasive cancer that is confined to the milk ducts and has not yet spread to the breast tissue. When DCIS is confined to a portion of the breast, it may be treated with breast-saving surgery; but when it spreads throughout the breast, mastectomy is the best treatment. A large invasive cancer—that is, a large tumor that has spread outside the ducts—may necessitate mastectomy in which a significant amount of skin may be taken along with the nipple and areola. Usually smaller invasive cancers accompanied by extensive DCIS or large, pure DCIS can be treated with skin-sparing mastectomy in concert with immediate reconstruction.

Skin-Sparing Modified Radical Mastectomy Before Breast Reconstruction

Skin-sparing mastectomy can be highly advantageous to the woman who desires reconstructive surgery immediately after mastectomy because the skin can be used as an envelope for a breast implant, latissimus flap, or TRAM flap (a type of reconstruction done with your own abdominal soft tissue, skin, and fat. See Chapter 9, "State-of-the-Art Breast Reconstruction.") Many studies have shown that the selected use of skin-sparing mastectomy yields survival rates that are equivalent to mastectomy in which the skin is taken. Thus, there is good data that skin-sparing mastectomy is an excellent option in certain situations, and we are continuing to see more data that is suggestive of how much skin can be saved while maintaining a low risk of local recurrence. There is always some risk that an invasive tumor could recur in the remaining skin, even when a lot of skin is removed. That's why the use of skin-sparing mastectomy requires a great deal of expertise and judgment and should be done only in situations where the chance that the tumor will come back in the skin is extremely low. The skin flaps must be thin, especially centrally, to assure the appropriate removal of the breast tissue.

If you have a tumor that is clearly far from the breast skin and the nipple/areolar complex, the breast skin and sometimes the areolar skin may be saved in selected cases. This is an area of recent, ongoing investigation and some controversy. However, I am increasingly but cautiously saving the areolar skin in my practice. The pathologist must look closely under the microscope to make sure that the cancer is nowhere near the nipple/areola complex on both frozen and permanent section. If the frozen section is suspicious, the areola skin is completely removed immediately. If the frozen section is negative, but the permanent pathology comes back positive, I reschedule my patient for removal of the areola at another time. Removing the areola is an outpatient procedure. If it is safe, many women want to preserve the areola for cosmetic and psychological reasons. We continue to follow these patients closely and have had no skin recurrences in this select population to date.

If you are a candidate for skin-sparing mastectomy, you must have a full discussion with your surgeon before surgery to find out about your surgeon's experience and results with skin-sparing mastectomy, the current direction of clinically acceptable practice, and the individual risks and benefits in your particular case before embarking on the procedure. Ask to talk to the doctor's patients who have had skin-sparing mastectomy and ask for the doctor's recurrence rates in the remaining skin of the breast over time and complication rates for skin sloughing, or dead skin, after surgery. Your doctor's rate of recurrence in the skin should be less than 5 percent, although clinical research is still ongoing in this area.

Prophylactic Bilateral Total Mastectomy

In very rare instances, a woman might be a candidate for a bilateral prophylactic total mastectomy (usually with immediate reconstruction), which entails removing both breasts. Taking out the majority of breast tissue can significantly reduce the likelihood of developing breast cancer for those patients who are appropriate candidates. Those highly-motivated individuals who may be included in the small group of potential candidates for bilateral prophylactic mastectomies are:

- Women who are BRCA-1 or BRCA-2 positive. (BRCA stands for breast cancer associated gene.) If you are positive for BRCA-1 or BRCA-2, you should be counseled about all of your treatment options.

- Women with *several* first-generation relatives who have breast cancer. This means first-degree relatives such as your mother, sister, or daughter.

- Women who have had *many* breast biopsies and continue to form lumps or suspicious mammographic lesions, especially when atypia or (lobular carcinoma in situ) LCIS has been diagnosed on prior biopsies. These are pathologic diagnoses in prior biopsies that increase the risk of developing breast cancer in the future.

- Women with extremely severe fibrocystic disease unresponsive to medical therapy. I am not referring to women with normal fibrocystic breasts but rather to women whose breasts are extremely painful, hard and lumpy and who often have uninterpretable mammograms. In these cases, it is very difficult to examine one's breasts for possible breast cancer with any degree of assuredness.

Prophylactic bilateral total mastectomy is not a modified radical mastectomy and does not entail lymph node removal nor does it entail removal of the nipple/areola complex. It can be followed by immediate breast reconstruction. I have rarely suggested prophylactic mastectomies with reconstruction and have talked many patients out of pursuing this procedure because they didn't need it. The determination to do this surgery can happen if the woman strongly wants it coupled with extensive discussion with her surgeon. Usually a patient requests this form of surgery after long consideration on her part.

Very few women are actually candidates for this procedure, and the surgeon assisting the woman interested in the surgery must make certain that she does not have cancer already. She should have a good physical examination, a mammogram preoperatively, and may also require ultrasound preoperatively.

- If at the time of the surgery a previously undetected cancer is noted on frozen section, the surgeon must make sure that the margins are clear and that appropriate lymph nodes are removed at the time. If the pathologist's initial impression is that the breast does not contain cancer, but a small cancer is found on permanent section, the margins will have to be assessed and the patient may be rescheduled for appropriate lymph node dissection.

After having faced the stress and trauma of several lumpectomies, two more lumps appeared in my breasts. At this point, I began to consider this very selective surgery. My surgeon and I discussed the possibility through the course of a year. He told me that it was not a guarantee that I would not get cancer and that there was a long recovery process; however, with no breast tissue, there was a 90 percent chance that I would not get another lump. I did a lot of research into my options, although it was difficult to find other women who had had this type of surgery. I vis-ited a plastic surgeon, and we determined that an implant reconstruction would be the best choice for me. Although my recovery was long and painful, I would do it again because I have peace of mind now. I would advise any woman who is considering this type of surgery to really take a look at herself before doing it and to do it for herself and no one else, to think about her options, and do her research. My left and right breasts do not look the same, but that's okay. This is a decision I made for my health, not out of vanity. You will need support through all of this. You will need family support, support from your significant other or partner, and support from other women who have been through this. I had a friend who had had a mastectomy with reconstruction and who helped me through the process and told me what to expect. • Josie

CHAPTER EIGHT

Removing Lymph Nodes

By Seth P. Harlow, M.D.

According to our current knowledge of breast cancers, all tumors that have an invasive component have the potential to spread (metastasize) to other sites in the body. Breast cancer cells can spread to distant organs through the bloodstream or through the lymphatic system to the lymph nodes. We can usually detect the spread of cancer to the lymph nodes before there is overt evidence of metastases to distant organs. Your risk of metastatic disease is related to the size of your tumor and the level of aggressiveness in the type of cancer that you have.

Lymphatic fluid from the breast drains primarily to the lymph nodes in the axilla (armpit region). The lymph nodes are small glands that are part of your immune system and help to protect you from bacteria, viruses, and other microorganisms. However, lymphatic flow from the breast can occasionally lead to lymph nodes outside the axilla, including nodes located just behind the ribs near the sternum (breastbone) called the *internal mammary lymph nodes*; just above the clavicle (collarbone) called *supraclavicular lymph nodes*; and within the breast itself called *intra-mammary lymph nodes*. Although lymphatic flow from a tumor can drain to any of these sites, in most people the axillary lymph nodes are the primary location to which a tumor drains. While breast cancer will usually spread first to the lymph nodes, breast cancer cells can spread to distant organ sites without there being evidence of metastatic disease in the regional lymph nodes. Because of this possibility, current recommendations provide for adjuvant systemic treatments (chemotherapy and hormonal therapy) for many patients with node negative breast cancers, although patients with very tiny cancers, or cancers that are very slow growing, and elderly patients may not receive chemotherapy.

Why Remove the Lymph Nodes? A Brief History

Until the 1970s, local treatment for breast cancer was based on Dr. William Halsted's teachings that breast cancer would progress by direct extension of the tumor through the lymphatic channels to the regional lymph nodes. It was thought that cancer could enter the bloodstream and metastasize to distant organ sites only after the cancer reached the lymph nodes. This theory served as the basis for the Halsted radical mastectomy in which the breast, chest wall muscles, and all the axillary (armpit) lymph nodes were removed to completely encompass all of the cancer. When it was later discovered that breast cancer cells actually reached the lymph nodes by migrating individually from the tumor site rather than by direct extension, the Halsted model was modified. But, with the exception of the introduction of the modified radical mastectomy, the overall goals for treatment didn't change, as it was still believed that cancer spread to

> Cancer cells can spread through the lymph system or bloodstream. Cancer in the lymph nodes can indicate whether the disease has spread (or metastasized). The spread of cancer can be detected in the lymph nodes before it is found in distant organs.

the lymph nodes before spreading to other areas of the body. During this period, surgeons who were disappointed with the high recurrence of disease in patients with lymph node metastases started experimenting with even more radical operations called extended radical mastectomies, in which the surgeon performed a radical mastectomy with removal of additional lymph nodes in the internal mammary lymph node chain. Because it was known that breast cancer could metastasize to this site, the hope was that this additional surgery could cure more patients. But these extensive procedures produced significant side effects, and when it was ultimately shown that they offered no survival benefits over standard radical mastectomies, they were abandoned.

It wasn't until the work of Dr. Bernard Fisher and colleagues in the latter half of the twentieth century that the Halsted model of breast cancer progression was challenged. Dr. Fisher conducted studies evaluating the blood of patients with breast and colorectal cancers and was able to identify circulating tumor cells in the bloodstream of many patients with early disease, even those without lymph node metastases. Fisher theorized that breast cancer cells could metastasize via the lymphatic pathways or the bloodstream at the same time and that this could happen at very early stages of the disease. He saw the regional lymph nodes simply as indicators of disease spread, positing that if metastatic disease were to be found in these nodes, cancer would inevitably be seen at distant organ sites. For Fisher, the presence of distant organ metastases was the ultimate determinant of patient survival, thus he suggested that less aggressive local-regional treatments would not alter patients' survival rates. Fisher was also the first surgeon to use evidence from prospective randomized clinical trials to justify his theories of breast cancer progression.

The prospective randomized clinical trial system developed to serve as an unbiased, scientifically valid method for comparing treatment options and has been widely applied to different cancer treatments. Dr. Fisher's clinical trial organization, the National Surgical Adjuvant Breast and Bowel Project (NSABP), performed two large surgical trials, the NSABP B-04 trial and the NSABP B-06 trial. The B-04 trial compared different methods of treatment of the axillary lymph nodes. Every patient in this study had a total mastectomy, but patients were randomized to have their lymph nodes treated either by surgical removal (called *axillary nodal dissection*), radiotherapy, or no treatment at all. The overall findings of this study indicated that there was no statistically significant difference in patient survival between these treatment options. The B-06 trial later extended these findings when women were randomized to receive a modified radical mastectomy; lumpectomy and axillary node dissection; or a lumpectomy, axillary dissection, and radiation. As with the B-04 trial, there were no statistically significant differences in patient survival in any of these treatment groups, and the findings of the B-06 trial have been confirmed in other prospective randomized trials of breast-saving surgery.

Although the B-04 trial didn't show a statistically significant difference in survival rates with axillary nodal observation versus treatment, the standard of care regarding the regional lymph nodes didn't change, because axillary dissection was the only treatment option that could reliably achieve the three goals of regional disease treatment, including:

• **Staging of the cancer.** We can only determine whether cancer has spread to the regional lymph nodes by surgical removal and microscopic evaluation. Nodal staging is the most important predictor of patient survival and is an integral part of the staging system for breast cancer. Lymph nodes and tumor size are the most important of several factors used to stage cancer. (For more information about staging, see Chapter 10, "Chemotherapy, Hormone Therapy, and the Stages of Breast Cancer.") The status of your lymph nodes is also the most important consideration used when making decisions about systemic adjuvant therapies, such as chemotherapy and hormone therapy. However, a patient can have metastatic cancer without having positive nodes, and adjuvant therapy may be recommended for a patient without positive nodes.

• **Regional disease control.** Cancer cells that are left in place in the regional nodes have the potential to grow within those nodes and eventually invade surrounding structures. This can lead to arm and chest pain due to invasion of adjacent nerves and arm swelling due to obstruction of the blood vessels and lymphatics in the arm. Results from clinical trials, including the NSABP B-04 trial, have shown that nodal recurrences affect 20 to 30 percent of patients who do not have their lymph nodes treated. When patients have their lymph node removed by axillary dissection, the regional recurrence rate is 1 to 3 percent.

• **Survival benefit.** Further scrutiny of the B-04 trials as well as the results of other similar studies have left some doubt about the original conclusions that there was not a survival difference between observed patients and those who had axillary treatment. As was previously mentioned, all patients in the B-04 trial had a total mastectomy. During this procedure, breast tissue extending into the axilla (armpit), the axillary tail of the breast, is routinely removed. It's very common to remove some of the lower axillary lymph nodes with the breast tissue during this part of the surgical procedure. These lymph nodes are frequently the first nodes where metastatic disease is found. In the B-04 trial, these low axillary nodes were removed and identified in approximately one-third of patients randomized to nodal observation. Tumor metastases were discovered in many of these cases, the removal of which might have improved the survival rate in this group compared to those patients who were truly observed. In addition, the B-04 trial found that patients who had their nodes treated, either by radiation or surgery, did in fact have more favorable survival rates. But this survival advantage was of such a small magnitude (4 to 5 percent improvement) that it failed to reach a level of statistical significance. Unfortunately, the number of patients enrolled in this trial was not great enough to have the statistical power to demonstrate significance to any survival difference less than seven percent. This lack of statistical power implies that survival differences greater than 7 percent are quite unlikely, but a true survival difference that is less than this number cannot be excluded based on the results of this study alone. A recent review of the world's literature found six prospective randomized clinical trials comparing axillary treatment to axillary observation in patients with invasive breast cancer. Using a method called *meta-analysis*, the results of these studies were combined, giving more than 3,000 patients for analysis. This meta-analysis demonstrated that a statistically significant survival benefit of approximately 5 percent was seen in patients receiving axillary treatment compared to observation. While this survival benefit may not be overly impressive, it is in the same range of overall survival benefit seen for patients receiving adjuvant systemic treatments for node negative disease and, when looked at in the context of the 180,000 women who develop breast cancer annually in the United States, may account for several thousand patients' lives being saved by adequate axillary treatment.

Given these potential advantages of axillary dissection, the National Cancer Institute issued guidelines in 1990 recommending a level 1 and 2 axillary lymph node dissection (removal of a number of axillary lymph nodes) as the optimum treatment for patients with invasive breast cancer.

Complications of Axillary Node Dissection and the Search for a Better Method

While axillary dissection does achieve the three goals of regional disease treatment, it does so at the expense of increased complications after surgery, including:

- Arm and chest wall lymphedema (swelling of the soft tissues), which occurs in about 5 to 30 percent of patients; and

- Upper arm numbness, pain, and decreased range of motion.

These problems are so common that axillary dissection is generally considered the most difficult part of breast cancer surgery, and because of these drawbacks, doctors have been looking for alternatives to axillary dissection for the past ten to fifteen years. A myriad of imaging modalities have been investigated, including axillary ultrasound, CT scanning, Magnetic Resonance Imaging (MRI), sestamibi nuclear scanning, and PET scanning, to find out if any of these noninvasive modalities could accurately identify patients with metastatic disease in the regional nodes. Unfortunately all of these modalities have been limited by one weakness, the inability to accurately identify small foci (tiny microscopic collections of cancer cells) of metastatic disease in the regional nodes. To date, these small collections of cancer cells can only be accurately detected by the pathologic evaluation of surgically removed lymph nodes.

The Sentinel Node Concept: Is It a Better Method?

Surgeons and students of anatomy began experimenting with mapping of the lymphatic pathways in the early to mid twentieth century. These early studies were usually done to identify all potential nodal drainage sites from a tumor, so that they could be included in surgical removal of that cancer. It wasn't until the 1970s that surgeons contemplated the notion of mapping the lymph nodes to identify the first draining lymph nodes. Dr. Ramon Cabanas, a urologic surgeon, was the first to test the hypothesis that the chief lymph node to drain a tumor site, a node he termed the *sentinel lymph node*, could predict the presence of tumor metastases to the regional lymph node basin. He performed sentinel node biopsy followed by a complete inguinal (groin) node dissection in a hundred patients with squamous cell carcinoma of the penis. The sentinel node predicted the presence or absence of tumor spread in all one hundred patients. But Cabanas's sentinel node concept didn't gain widespread attention until the early 1990s when Dr. Donald Morton described a lymphatic mapping and sentinel lymph node biopsy procedure in melanoma that had a similarly high rate of pathologic correlation to a complete lymph node dissection (98 percent). After his report, the interest in sentinel node biopsy procedures for other cancer types rose dramatically, with its use in breast cancer gaining the most popularity.

> The sentinel node (or nodes) is the chief node to drain a tumor site and is the lymph node most likely to contain cancer. It can predict the presence of cancer spread to the lymph node basin.

Sentinel Lymph Node Biopsy in Breast Cancer: Two Ways to Detect the Sentinel Node

There are two preferred methods by which surgeons detect the sentinel lymph node in breast cancer: the blue dye lymphatic mapping technique and a gamma probe guided radiolabeled tracer technique. Both have unique advantages and disadvantages and have been extensively studied.

Blue Dye Lymphatic Mapping

Initially described by Dr. Armando Guiliano and colleagues, this procedure employs a small volume of a blue dye (isosulfan blue dye or patent blue V dye) injected directly into the breast tissue around the site of the breast cancer. The blue dye enters the lymphatic channels and is transported to the first lymph node or nodes into which these channels drain. The surgeon makes an incision in the axilla (armpit region) and attempts to visually identify the blue-stained lymphatic channels. Once these channels are located, they are followed until they lead into a lymph node or nodes, which are generally stained blue as well. No radioactivity is used, and the blue dye reaches the sentinel nodes in a very short time. This allows the surgeon to perform the injection in the operating room after you have been anesthetized. There are potential disadvantages of this technique, including the fact that the exact location of the sentinel node cannot be determined until an incision is made. If this incision is not placed in an optimal location, the surgeon may have to dissect through a larger volume of normal tissue to identify the sentinel node. Additionally, once a sentinel node is identified and removed, the surgeon must confirm that no other sentinel nodes are present, as there often is more than one sentinel node. This may involve additional dissection of normal tissue that can lead to increased complications, the avoidance of which is the entire reason for doing the sentinel node biopsy in the first place.

Some of the known adverse effects of the blue dye include:

• Risk of skin tattooing at the injection site, which is rare.

• Blue-green urine for one to two days, which is common.

• Generalized blue discoloration of skin that lasts one or two days, which is uncommon.

• Allergic reaction to the dye can vary in severity but may require medical intervention. These allergic reactions occur in just under one percent of patients undergoing these procedures.

The Gamma Probe–Guided Radiolabeled Technique

Dr. David Krag at the University of Vermont first described the use of radiolabeled tracers and a handheld gamma probe to identify sentinel lymph nodes. In this technique, a radioactive tracer is injected into the breast around the tumor. This tracer migrates through the lymphatic channels to the sentinel nodes, where it becomes trapped. The surgeon uses a small handheld gamma detector probe in a sterile sheath to identify the lymph nodes before making any incision, thereby minimizing the odds of having to cut through significant amounts of normal tissue. Once the sentinel nodes are removed, the surgeon can verify that all sentinel nodes have been excised simply by confirming with the gamma probe that no additional areas of radioactivity remain. The radiolabeled method can also identify sentinel lymph nodes outside the axilla, which include the nodes between the ribs near the sternum, above the collarbone, and inside the breast itself. Five to 20 percent of patients have sentinel nodes in these areas, and they may be sites of metastatic spread. These nodes are not routinely removed in breast cancer treatment, although they rarely may be the only sites of tumor spread in some people. They are not evaluated with the blue dye technique because this would require that the surgeon explore each of these areas looking for the blue dye when in fact lymphatic drainage to these sites occurs in only a small percentage of patients.

The disadvantages of the radiolabel technique include the need for the radioactive tracer, which requires specific handling to comply with hospital radiation safety guidelines and the use of specialized equipment—the gamma probe—which has cost and training issues associated with it. The typical dose of radioactivity used for sentinel node procedures is one millicurie or less, which amounts to less radioactivity exposure than a standard chest X ray. From the procedural standpoint, the typical radiolabeled tracer (technetium sulfur colloid) must be injected at least 30 minutes before surgery, outside of the operating room while you are awake. The timing of the injection is critical to finding the sentinel node rather than additional nonsentinel nodes, which will eventually take up the radiolabeled tracer. Injections typically cause minor pain that lasts about five minutes. Allergic reactions to these agents are quite rare and are much less frequent than with the blue dye. There are potential technical problems for the surgeon using this method as there can be overlap of radioactivity from the breast injection site if it is near the likely lymph node locations. These problems, however, can be overcome with proper use of the probe in almost all such cases and should rarely prevent accurate sentinel node identification.

The Risk of False Negatives in Sentinel Node Biopsy

In the past decade, a number of authors have published results defining the accuracy of sentinel lymph node biopsy in breast cancer. In all of these studies, the sentinel lymph nodes were removed along with the remaining axillary lymph nodes in an axillary dissection. The pathologic status of the sentinel lymph nodes was then compared to the

A false negative occurs when all sentinel nodes are negative and a node from the remaining axillary dissection has cancer.

pathologic status of the entire axillary dissection. The results of all the published studies have been quite similar. Sentinel lymph nodes can be identified in 80 to 90 percent of patients, and the pathologic accuracy rate of the sentinel nodes in predicting the regional lymph node status is 95 to 100 percent. However, when we employ a more rigorous evaluation of the accuracy of sentinel lymph node biopsy, with the determination of the false negative rate, these procedures carry a 0 to 15 percent risk of providing false information. Determining the false neg-

BLUE DYE AND RADIOLABELED TECHNIQUES WORK BEST IN COMBINATION

An evaluation of the different methods and techniques shows that, in most surgeons' hands, a combination of the blue dye and radiolabeled methods offers the highest chance of locating the sentinel nodes and accurately determining the presence of metastases in those nodes. The surgeon who uses both methods at the same time has a second option for sentinel node identification in case one method fails. In addition, sentinel lymph nodes in sites outside the axilla should be removed, as up to 10 percent of these may harbor metastatic disease and in a few cases this will be the only site of metastatic disease in a patient.

ative rate is important, because it tells us about true efficacy of a procedure. The false negative rate of this procedure is determined by how accurate the procedure is in identifying cancer in the lymph nodes when in fact there are lymph node metastases present somewhere in the regional lymph node basin. Where there are no lymph node metastases, any lymph node that is removed and tested will show the same result, whether it is truly the sentinel node or not. It is only when nodal metastases are present that the efficacy of the technique can be judged.

Hidden Metastatic Disease

Before sentinel lymph node biopsy procedures, most pathologists evaluated the axillary nodes from an axillary dissection in a rather limited fashion. This was primarily because an axillary dissection specimen would usually include 10 to 25 lymph nodes and to perform an exhaustive evaluation of each of these nodes was not feasible from a time and cost perspective. In the era of sentinel node biopsy, however, the pathologist is handed a small number of lymph nodes known to be the ones most likely to contain metastatic disease. They can now expend a greater amount of effort on this limited number of nodes and potentially identify metastatic disease that might otherwise be missed with standard evaluations, the so-called *occult (hidden) metastatic disease*. Techniques used to find hidden evidence of cancer spread include:

> **THE VALUE OF SENTINEL NODE BIOPSY**
>
> Sentinel node biopsy can identify the lymph node(s) most likely to contain cancer and can decrease the potential complications of more aggressive axillary node dissections. The smaller number of lymph nodes pathologists are given to examine allows pathologists to concentrate on finding hidden metastatic disease, using serial sectioning and, currently in clinical trials, IHC staining.

- **Serial sectioning.** Multiple sections of the lymph node are cut and put on slides to be evaluated by standard staining methodology. Because more of the node is visualized, the chance of identifying small tumor deposits is increased.

• **Immunohistochemical (IHC) staining.** In recent years, newer methods of staining tumor cells using monoclonal antibodies targeting specific proteins produced by cancer cells have been developed. The most common antibodies used for breast cancer are those that recognize cellular proteins called cytokeratins, which are produced by almost all breast cancer cells. These techniques are incredibly sensitive as individual tumor cells can easily be identified in a background of nonmalignant lymph node cells. The problem with these techniques, however, is that they may be too sensitive and may identify clinically meaningless isolated tumor cells that have migrated to the lymph node during the surgical procedure or the breast biopsy, have no potential to grow in the lymph node, and thus may not be representative of true metastatic disease.

Both of these methods will identify disease that may otherwise be missed with standard pathologic evaluation. It is clear, however, that the IHC methods have the greatest potential to provide false information regarding a patient's need for adjuvant therapies like chemotherapy and hormone therapy. A recent consensus conference by the College of American Pathologists has issued a statement saying that IHC techniques should not be used in the standard evaluation of sentinel lymph nodes but rather should be restricted to clinical trials until its predictive value is demonstrated. The prognostic significance of occult metastases is a critical part of the two ongoing sentinel lymph node studies.

Clinical Trials: Axillary Lymph Node Dissection Versus Sentinel Node Biopsy

As we've seen, sentinel lymph node biopsy procedures have been found to be very accurate predictors of cancer spread to the regional lymph nodes in patients with invasive breast cancer, but still have a documented false negative rate of up to 15 percent. To date, there have been no definitive studies comparing sentinel node biopsy alone to an axillary dissection, which is still considered the standard treatment. The National Cancer Institute has recently sponsored two large prospective randomized clinical trials to evaluate the safety and effectiveness of sentinel node biopsy compared to standard surgical treatments.

The first trial, being run by the University of Vermont through the NSABP clinical trials group, is the NSABP B-32 trial. In this trial, eligible patients who consent to enroll will be randomized to one of two treatment groups. Group 1 patients will have a sentinel node biopsy procedure performed followed by a completion axillary node dissection. This group is considered the standard surgery arm, as all patients will have a level 1 and 2 lymph node dissection. The sentinel node procedure is added to this group because the sentinel nodes may be located outside the axilla in 5 to 15 percent of cases, which would otherwise be missed with a standard axillary dissection. Group 2 patients will have a sentinel node biopsy performed but will only have an axillary dissection if metastatic disease is found in the sentinel nodes. All patients will be assessed for time to disease recurrence and length of survival. Additional measurements of arm mobility, sensory changes, and arm edema (swelling) will be assessed and compared between groups. The B-32 study is anticipated to include 5,400 patients, giving this study adequate statistical power to detect as little as a 2 percent difference in survival between the two study arms. This study should give the definitive answer to the safety of this procedure in patients with pathologically negative sentinel nodes.

The second trial is being run through the American College of Surgeons Oncology Group (ACOSOG) in its Z0011 trial. To be eligible for this trial, a patient will need to have had a sentinel node biopsy that has demonstrated the presence of metastatic disease. Eligible patients who give informed consent will be randomized to a standard treatment arm of a completion axillary dissection versus a study arm of no further surgery. Patients will be followed in a similar fashion as the B-32 study for time to recurrence and length of survival. This study will determine the validity of the original Fisher hypothesis that lymph node metastases are indicators and not determinants of patient outcome and will complete our knowledge base on the need for regional node dissection in people with breast cancer.

It is the current recommendation of the National Cancer Institute that the use of sentinel lymph node biopsy alone as a treatment for invasive breast cancer should not be considered as a standard of care in this disease until the results of these two trials are reported. They also encourage all eligible patients to participate in either of these trials, or other similar trials, that may further evaluate the efficacy and safety of sentinel node techniques.

My surgeon told me that he had removed two lymph nodes. He had explained to me earlier that he would do this to make sure the cancer had not spread. They were positive for cancer, so he had removed 14 all together. • Cynthia

Sentinel node biopsy is only as good as the person doing it. Ask how many times he or she has done the procedure before. You may have to go to a teaching hospital or medical center, but do it. My sister had a full axillary node dissection and she has a problem with lymphedema. Sentinel node biopsy can be a wonderful tool to cut down on problems associated with axillary lymph node dissection. • Anne

The Gold Standard for Treatment of the Lymph Nodes

It is tempting to use the encouraging preliminary results of sentinel lymph node biopsy procedures to justify the abandonment of routine axillary dissection for treatment of invasive breast cancer. These techniques identify metastatic disease very accurately with significantly less tissue removal and thus fewer complications for patients after surgery. The current NSABP and ACOSOG clinical trials will give definitive answers about the safety and efficacy of these procedures and will define when and where they can be used as stand-alone procedures in the future. The final results from the NSABP trial will be available in 2004 to 2005. The ACOSOG trial may take longer to be completed.

But sentinel lymph node biopsy does have a role in treatment today.

SENTINEL NODE BIOPSY AND DCIS

The role of sentinel node biopsy in ductal carcinoma in situ (DCIS) is not clear at the present. Some studies have shown metastases in sentinel lymph nodes in DCIS, but these have usually only been by IHC and may not be of clinical significance. Because the number of patients in these studies is very small, further studies are needed.

| ARE YOU A CANDIDATE FOR SENTINEL NODE BIOPSY?

Currently we recommend sentinel node biopsy and axillary lymph node dissection as the standard of care, although many surgeons are doing sentinel node biopsy alone based on preliminary studies. The question of whether to do sentinel node biopsy alone or in conjunction with axillary node dissection is a matter for each patient and doctor to decide. However, patients selected for sentinel node biopsy should have:

• Unifocal breast cancer (only one cancer in the breast)

• Clinically uninvolved axillary lymph nodes (negative nodes); and

• No evidence of metastases.

Any patient with invasive breast cancer should be considered a potential candidate for axillary dissection. Patients with other medical conditions that place them at high surgical risk or who have a limited amount of life expectancy may not be good candidates for sentinel node biopsy or axillary lymph node dissection.

Because sentinel node biopsy procedures have the potential to identify sentinel nodes outside the axilla that may contain metastatic disease and because serial sectioning may identify small but clinically meaningful deposits of metastatic disease, sentinel node biopsy followed by additional axillary node dissection should be considered the new gold standard in the management of invasive breast cancer. This will ensure patients the most comprehensive evaluation and treatment of regional lymph nodes that is available. While other management strategies may equal this treatment, none would exceed it for regional disease control and patient survival. We all hope that the current clinical trials will prove that sentinel node biopsy alone will be as safe as standard surgery. We will then be able to decrease side effects of surgery while knowing that are we not adversely affecting survival.

Does Your Surgeon Have the Expertise to Perform These Surgeries?

This is a matter of some controversy, but most surgeons and the Society of Breast Surgeons generally agree that a surgeon will need to have done about 20 sentinel lymph node biopsies and axillary lymph node dissections in order to gain the necessary confidence to perform these procedures. Surgeons should be able to tell you their success rates at finding sentinel nodes as well as their false negative rates. Those surgeons who have undergone intensive training procedures, such as those needed to participate in the NSABP B-32 study, have shown similar success with both procedures after a smaller number of cases (five) as those with greater case numbers. For more information about choosing your surgeon, see Chapter 19, "How to Get the Best Care and Treatment."

CHAPTER NINE

State-of-the-Art Breast
Reconstruction

By J. Arthur Jensen, M.D., F.A.C.S.

There is in fact no gold standard of reconstruction because just as each woman is an individual so too is each reconstruction. While it's true that some kinds of reconstruction are better than others, they involve more extensive surgery, time, and cost. I encourage you to use this chapter not to determine what type of reconstruction is best, but to help you think about what type of reconstruction is best for you.

We'll look at two types of reconstruction, including flap reconstruction, which uses your own tissues to reconstruct your breast, and implant reconstruction, which uses materials that are not part of your body. Options for flap reconstruction include a latissimus dorsi flap (which uses back muscle and tissue) with or without an implant, or a TRAM flap (which uses lower abdominal muscle and tissue), and which requires no implant. Alternatively, women may choose implant reconstruction. This generally involves placing a tissue expander and then replacing it with a "permanent" implant. We will discuss the advantages and disadvantages of the various options shortly.

There are two guiding principles to consider when deciding what type of reconstruction is right for you.

What Value Do You Place on the Appearance of Your Breasts?

All women do not value their breasts equally. So the first question you must ask yourself is how important your breast is to you. Your breasts may be terribly important to your social, psychological, and sexual life, or you may simply wish to look more "balanced" in clothing. While generalizations might be made about the meaning of one's breast during any given period of life, every woman must be treated as an individual. I have performed the most advanced flap procedures on women in their seventies. Conversely, I have met women in their fifties who have little interest in the appearance of their breast. You alone must approach the question of reconstruction with a personal understanding of how important your breast is to your well-being.

All Reconstructions Are Not the Same

Some reconstructive techniques leave an almost normal breast while others leave only a crude approximation. The choices a woman and her treating doctors make at the time of mastectomy determine how good the final result will be. To some extent, these decisions are made on the basis of what kind of breast cancer a woman has and how advanced the cancer is at the time of discovery.

When the skin of the breast can be saved from removal, a reconstruction can almost look as good as the original. But when the skin must be taken for cancer reasons, the burden of reconstruction is clearly very different because there is no skin to serve as an envelope for an implant or a flap, making natural reconstruction very unlikely.

Mastectomy is the removal of the breast gland. Many surgeons consider removal of the nipple and areola (the dark skin around the nipple) to be part of any "good" mastectomy. Furthermore, some surgeons insist that removing an ellipse of skin around the areola is also important to prevent recurrence of cancer. However, there is a growing realization among cancer surgeons that previous assumptions about breast cancer treatment should be reexamined. When breast cancer involves the skin, clearly the skin must be removed. But often, the cancer does not involve the skin and there is no reason to compromise a woman's final aesthetic result by removing healthy skin. If the breast skin can be spared, then only the mass of the breast needs to be reconstructed. This maximizes the chance of a truly "normal" reconstruction.

Most of the women I've talked to had TRAM flaps. But implants are also available. Each option has a certain amount of pain associated with it, and the pain can be excruciating for a brief period of time. I think it's important to know exactly what type of operation you are having, exactly how much pain you will be in, as well as the pros and cons of your options for pain control. • Joelle

Even when I wear a bathing suit, I feel comfortable. I am more confident. When my reconstruction was first done, it was very hard, but as time went on, it grew softer and hung like my other breast. It's been wonderful. I couldn't be happier. My breast isn't the same. Your body isn't the same, but to wake up from surgery and see a mound on my chest meant everything to me. When I see my scars, I don't say, "Oh, how ugly." I say, "Without these scars, I wouldn't be here." And the scars appear less and less prominent as time goes on. • Linda L.

Implant Reconstruction

There is no subject in the world of reconstructive surgery more controversial than that of breast implants. At the time of this writing, there is no evidence that breast implants cause systemic disease, as was alleged in the early 1990s. Multiple studies done by epidemiologists (medical specialists trained to examine such questions in population-based studies) have concluded that breast implants do have their problems, but that implants do not give women systemic illness.

Most implant reconstructions are done in stages. First, a deflated implant called a tissue expander is placed into a space beneath the muscles of the chest wall. Later, after the wounds heal, the tissue expander is filled with fluid, stretching the skin. This process can take weeks to months, and is generally done in-office. It may hurt a bit, but no anesthetic is necessary. Finally, the tissue expander is removed and replaced with a "permanent" implant. Using tissue expanders and implants is the most common technique performed for breast reconstruction today. There is no need to involve any other area of a woman's body, as in flap reconstruction where there is a need to harvest material to reconstruct the breast. In other words, the tissue expander and the implant come out of a box and are designed for safe implantation. A second advantage is that the time required to perform an implant is relatively short. A tissue expander can be placed under the muscles of the chest wall (the pectoralis major and the serratus anterior) in approximately an hour or less. Third, most plastic surgeons have the training and expertise to perform this procedure in a community hospital. Obviously, some surgeons will have more expertise than others in performing breast reconstruction but most have experience with implant reconstruction. Finally, the recovery period for an implant reconstruction is relatively short compared with flap reconstruction. Most women's wounds will heal and they will be back to their usual activities by three to four weeks.

Disadvantages of Implant Reconstruction

Implants also have their disadvantages. Although better than previous technologies, today's breast implant is not perfect. This is an important point and worthy of repeating. In the past, many surgeons told their patients that implants were essentially indestructible and would be trouble-free. Unfortunately, this is simply not true. There are problems with implants, and every woman who agrees to get an implant must understand what they are and how likely they are to occur.

Problems with implants can be divided into categories, including early problems, such as bleeding or infection; immediate problems, such as capsular contracture; and late problems, such as leakage of the saline or silicone and the need for future operations.

• **Bleeding and infection** can complicate all operations, no matter how small. Although there is only a slight risk of these complications, every patient can bleed and every patient can get infected. In my practice, the chances that bleeding and infection will complicate an implant reconstruction are less than one in a hundred. Flap procedures also carry risk of bleeding and infection, and some surgeons might say that the risk is even higher in these procedures. I believe that the risk of bleeding or infection is so low with either procedure that it shouldn't be a basis of one's decision for reconstruction.

• **Capsular contracture.** The biggest problem with implants is the buildup of scar tissue around the implant, which can make the implant feel firm and, in some cases, hard. It's not the implant that's hard; it will always be soft. The scar tissue around the implant tightens and makes the implant feel hard. A breast implant that feels firm is referred to as having *capsular contracture* whether in a reconstructive or elective augmentation. (The scar tissue around the implant is called the *capsule*. When the scar tissue tightens around the implant making it hard or painful, it's said to be contracted.) Plastic surgeons have struggled with capsular contracture for decades. It doesn't always occur, and it's hard to have an understanding of how it occurs. Our studies at the Breast Center in Van Nuys demonstrated that the longer we followed women with breast implants, the more capsular contacture we observed. When patients were followed for five years, approximately 30 to 40 percent could be expected to get firm breast implants. Clearly, the risk of capsular contracture increases over time.

Surgery is the only treatment for capsular contracture, although a woman may have a mild contracture that does not require surgery. In the procedure to treat a capsular contracture, the breast implant is exposed, the capsule around the implant is removed, and the same or another implant is placed in the dissected pocket. Usually, this isn't a terribly difficult procedure, and it is well within the experience and expertise of most plastic surgeons.

If you choose implants, you must be aware that capsular contracture is a possibility and that the likelihood of this complication increases over time. Understanding these limitations is part of informed consent.

How Will My Breast Feel after Implant Reconstruction?

Every woman who undergoes mastectomy loses some sensation in the breast skin because the nerves to the skin go through the breast gland itself and are cut during mastectomy. Sensation improves somewhat over time. A breast that has been reconstructed with an implant often feels to the touch like the underlying implant. If the implant is made with a silicone gel (that is, a silicone shell on the outside filled with a viscous silicone gel on the inside), an implant can feel very breastlike. A saline-filled implant (a silicone shell on the outside filled with saltwater on the inside) does not feel normal because the saline does not have the same softness as breast tissue or silicone gel. I prefer saltwater (saline) implants, because I find most women don't trust silicone gel in their bodies, and most of my patients are happy with saline implants. Occasionally a woman will be dissatisfied with the external feel of the implant and will ask to be switched over to gel.

Saline versus Silicone Implants: Pros and Cons

If an implant leaks, the body is further exposed to the material inside. Saltwater implants contain the same kind of liquid as in intravenous solutions used during any operation. There does not seem to be any serious threat to a patient's health when a saltwater implant leaks. The worse case scenario would require the placement of another implant. Silicone gel implants contain a viscous formulation of silicone, which can escape into the body. Unlike saline implants, a gel implant does not deflate when it leaks, and often goes undetected. The gel can go to the tissues around the implant. Occasionally silicone gel will be found in the lymph nodes of a patient with silicone gel implants. Although the medical community has no proof that this is harmful, no patient or doctor likes the idea of silicone appearing in a lymph node.

Safety issues regarding silicone gel have occupied the courts for at least a decade. Many patients prefer silicone implants because they feel more natural to the touch and are less likely to show any rippling through the skin. Women who are not happy with the feel of the saline implant or are significantly bothered by rippling may choose to have a gel implant, but must accept the risks, known and unknown, of this type of implant.

Radiation Therapy and Implants

Unfortunately, medicine is an imperfect science. Surgeons may feel that they are operating on a well-controlled cancer when they perform a mastectomy only to learn postoperatively that the cancer was more aggressive. Radiation therapy might be advised under these circumstances. Implant reconstruction does not tolerate radiation well. This adds yet another level of complexity to this choice, because the chances of capsular contracture following radiation therapy increase alarmingly.

That's why most plastic surgeons don't believe an implant should be used for someone who is known to need radiation. The risk that the implant will become hard and painful is so great that it is said to be

> If radiation will be a part of your treatment plan, implants may not be the right choice for you as implants do not tolerate radiation well.

contraindicated. Therefore, if radiation is likely to be necessary from the outset, a flap procedure without any implant is greatly preferable.

Patients sometimes ask if they can get radiation and then get an implant later so that the radiation does not make the implant firm. Unhappily, this is not the case. Radiation does not make implants firm; it has its effect on the surrounding tissue. As mentioned previously, it is the interaction between the implant and the surrounding tissue that makes the implant feel firm, as scar tissue builds up around the implant. The biological mechanisms that cause this problem are not fully known, but it is well recognized that patients who have been radiated do not tolerate implants as well as those who have not been radiated. If you are likely to need radiation therapy, you should carefully discuss with your plastic surgeon whether an implant reconstruction is advisable.

Choosing the Size and Shape of Your Implant

Breast implants come in different sizes and shapes. Every plastic surgeon has a bias about what kind of implant has worked best in that plastic surgeon's practice. If you do choose an implant, be sure to discuss possible implant types with your doctor before the operation that replaces the tissue expander with the implant.

Constructing the Nipple and Areola after Implant Reconstruction

The final stage of reconstruction is usually the reconstruction of the nipple/areolar complex. A patient must heal from her operation and be comfortable with the size, shape, and location of the implant before the final stage of breast reconstruction.

The nipple/areolar complex can be reconstructed in a number of ways. The nipple itself is usually reconstructed by designing small locally based flaps, which give an impression of a nipple. The tissue around the nipple flap can be tattooed or new skin can be taken from elsewhere on the body to provide the pigment needed by the areolar reconstruction. Reconstruction of the nipple/areolar complex is a relatively minor procedure and is commonly done as outpatient surgery.

After reconstruction of the nipple/areolar complex, most patients will feel as though their reconstruction is complete. However, I should stress that patient satisfaction is the endpoint of a reconstruction. Sometimes a woman will want a modification of a flap or placement of a larger or smaller implant. These kinds of modifications can be relatively minor and yet make a great difference to the way you feel about your surgery.

Flap Procedures

When a large piece of skin is transferred from one area of the body to another, it is said to be a *flap*. Skin grafts are very thin sheets of skin harvested from one area of the body and transferred without new blood supply to another area. For instance, it's possible to take skin from the leg and graft it to the breast. But this technique will work only with small amounts of skin. To move a significant amount of the body's fat requires that it be moved on a supply of blood. As you may know, all tissue relies on blood supply to bring in oxygen and nutrients to the tissue and to remove carbon dioxide and wastes. The greater the amount of tissue removed, the more blood supply is required for safe transfer. The flaps most frequently used in breast reconstruction come from the abdomen (the TRAM flap) or the back (latissimus dorsi flap). Tissues can be taken from other areas, such as the legs, but these procedures are less common.

The TRAM Flap

The transverse abdominal myocutaneous (TRAM) flap is the most common choice for complete autologous (own tissue) reconstruction. During the operation, skin and fat are moved from the lower abdomen and placed in the mastectomy defect (where the breast was removed). The tissue from the abdomen is mostly skin and fat and is thus an excellent replacement for the tissue removed by mastectomy. After a TRAM flap, the abdominal skin is significantly tighter, similar to a tummy tuck. Once the abdominal tissue heals in the mastectomy defect, the flap can feel almost identical to the unaffected breast. This is particularly true when the skin of the breast has been preserved.

Almost all plastic surgeons who specialize in breast reconstruction agree that autologous tissue reconstruction, when successfully done, gives the best long-term result.

If the TRAM flap gives such a natural result, why isn't it done in all cases? As mentioned previously, reconstruction of the breast mound with a tissue expander followed by an implant offers us the advantage of using man-made material. It doesn't need to be "harvested" from another area of the body. The TRAM flap must be removed from the abdomen and safely transferred to the chest wall with a reliable and adequate blood supply. It is a more technically demanding operation and involves risks that implants do not.

The early risks of the TRAM flap procedure are like the risks of implants—bleeding and infection. As a practical matter, neither of these risks is common. The biggest risk is whether the tissue will stay alive following its transfer to the chest wall. If a portion of the flap doesn't get enough blood supply, it will not live. When this happens, the tissue is said to be *necrotic*.

A successful TRAM flap transfer involves two basic variables: the surgeon's experience and the kind of transfer that is being done.

Single Muscle (Unipedicle) TRAM Flap

The large ellipse of skin and fat on the lower abdomen that is transferred as a TRAM flap needs a reliable blood supply. Fortunately, two muscles—the rectus abdomini—run up and down directly beneath this skin and fat. Arteries and veins run below these muscles, rise up and penetrate into the muscles, and then go from the muscles into the skin and fat that is attached to the muscles.

When first introduced, the TRAM flap was done by separating the skin and fat of the lower abdomen away from the surrounding tissues, but leaving it attached to one of the rectus muscles. This type of transfer is referred to as a *unipedicle TRAM flap* because it involves only one muscle. This sort of procedure involves lifting the fat and skin up on the underlying muscle and twisting the muscles so that the skin and fat end up in the mastectomy defect on the chest wall. Although this procedure can produce excellent results, it can also be complicated by insufficient blood supply to the fat and skin. If you smoke cigarettes, are overweight, or have had previous radiation therapy, you will not be considered a good candidate for this procedure as some necrosis or tissue damage is common in such patients (about 20 to 30 percent). When surgeons realized that this group had more tissue death or so called *necrosis,* they decided to move the skin and fat on both muscles and developed the bipedicle TRAM flap.

The Bipedicle TRAM Flap

The skin and fat of the lower abdomen can almost always be safely moved if both rectus muscles are sacrificed. But because both muscles have to be taken, this choice leaves a greater defect on the abdomen. Clearly, most women would rather have only one of the rectus muscles altered, if given a choice, so as to preserve the other rectus muscle. Long-term studies of abdominal muscle function show that patients return to their preoperative strength by about three months, regardless of what kind of flap they have.

The Free TRAM Flap

Another way to move tissue is to completely detach it from the body—in other words, free it—and then reattach it on the chest wall. This procedure involves reattaching the tissue flap's blood supply to blood vessels that run on the chest wall.

From a surgeon's perspective, it is not difficult to detach a flap from the body. The problem arises in reattaching it to the chest wall. It's not possible to simply sew the tissue to the chest wall because this does not bring adequate blood supply. For a free flap to work, the small arteries and veins that supply and drain the flap must be reattached to similar-sized vessels on the chest wall. The reattachment, or *anastomosis*, must be done under a microscope using special instruments and sutures. This is referred to as a *microvascular surgery*. Not all plastic surgeons are trained in this technique.

The free flap generally gives the best cosmetic result. The transferred tissue is not twisted, and the blood supply is generally completely reliable. Therefore, it rarely becomes hard (fat necrosis), and there is no bulge of tissue over the lower aspect of the rib cage where the muscle pedicle is twisted up to the chest wall as in a unipedicle or bipedicle TRAM flap. The other advantage to the free flap is that it is based on less muscle than a unipedicle flap. Only part of one muscle needs to be used to safely transfer the tissue. The disadvantage of the free flap is that not all plastic surgeons are trained to do this procedure and the operation can take many hours because of the microsurgery involved.

The Latissimus Dorsi Myocutaneous Flap

The latissimus dorsi is a muscle that runs beneath the skin of the posterior chest wall. It was the first muscle to be used for breast reconstruction. Skin and fat from the back can be centered on the latissimus dorsi muscle and transferred to the chest wall by rotating the muscle on its own blood supply. Twisted on its own blood supply, the muscle serves as the pedicle on which the skin and fat survive. Unlike the pedicle

The best breast reconstruction results occur when your breast surgeon and plastic surgeon work together and when reconstruction is performed immediately after mastectomy.

TRAM flap, the arc of rotation of the latissimus dorsi muscle is rather small, and the chance of compromising the blood supply is very low, even in heavy patients.

The problem with the latissimus dorsi flap is the limited amount of fat and skin that can be transferred. The fat deposit of the lower abdomen is much greater than the fat deposit over the back. Very often, there isn't enough tissue on the back that can be transferred to adequately reconstruct the breast, and an implant is usually required in addition to the flap to create the breast mound. Nevertheless, the latissimus flap is a very good choice for women with small breasts who don't require much tissue for reconstruction. It's also a reasonable choice to reconstruct the breast when a complete mastectomy is not necessary. (See Chapter 6, "Saving the Breast.") Even when used over an implant, the latissimus flap is a good choice for women who want a natural feel to the breast. The padding of the skin and fat from the back makes the implant much more natural to the touch.

The latissimus flap leaves a scar on the back, which is generally well-tolerated. My patients have less pain with the latissimus flap than they do with the TRAM flap, and they tend to leave the hospital around the third postoperative day. The wound on the back takes a couple of weeks to heal fully. I ask that patients do not drive for at least three weeks following the operation.

Recovering from TRAM Flap Surgery

The TRAM flap leaves a scar over the lower abdomen. My patients almost always leave the hospital on the fourth or fifth postoperative day. Everyone wants to drive by the fourteenth day, but I ask that they do not drive until the twenty-first day following the operation. Wanting to resume former activities, like driving, doesn't mean your wounds are healed, but this should give you an idea of how people feel two weeks after the operation.

AFTER YOUR SURGERY: CONTROLLING PAIN

There are many details regarding the postoperative course. Some patients are comfortable using a patient controlled analgesia (PCA) device in the days following the operation. This allows them to give themselves morphine or Demerol, as they need it. Some patients do not like this choice and want intramuscular injections of pain medicine. The details of your pain management will be individually tailored to your needs.

The way your breast will look immediately after surgery depends on how the mastectomy incision is made. If you have a skin-sparing mastectomy and all the mastectomy skin survives, the new breast can look very good from the outset. The nipple/areolar complex can be reconstructed after the flap has fully healed.

The Stages of Reconstruction

The nipple/areolar complex can be reconstructed after the breast mound has been reconstructed either by a tissue expander and an implant or by a flap. I prefer to do this procedure after the reconstruction of the breast mound rather than at the time of mastectomy, although some surgeons attempt to do everything at once. At the time that I reconstruct the nipple/areolar complex, I like to try to bring the opposite breast into symmetry. Sometimes this involves making the breast smaller, lifting the opposite breast, or in rare cases, making the opposite breast larger. In general, patients should think of this as a series of operations, or a staged process, as opposed to something that is done in a single day.

Choosing Your Plastic Surgeon

When choosing your plastic surgeon you should consider a few basic points:

• Your plastic surgeon should discuss all options available for reconstruction and should be competent to perform any of the procedures. If the surgeon can only perform an implant reconstruction, this will be your only choice.

• In addition, you might ask to see photographs of previous reconstructions performed by the plastic surgeon. Keep in mind that no plastic surgeon is going to show photographs of bad results, and yet results are not always consistently good. Ask to see a range of results from the plastic surgeon. Which results does he or she think are particularly good and which are bad?

| GETTING THE BEST RESULT

The quality of any breast reconstruction depends on:

- The amount of skin taken from the breast by the breast cancer surgeon

- The kind of material used to replace your breast—that is, an implant versus a flap reconstruction

- The experience of the plastic surgeon performing the operation

In addition, it is my deeply held belief that patients are best served if their doctors are willing to work together as a team. When I performed cancer surgery, I was always reluctant to encourage my patients to have reconstruction at the time of mastectomy because this invariably meant coordinating schedules between the oncologic team and the plastic surgical team. Everything became more complicated, and we all have a tendency to think of our own convenience. But having seen the difference in the results with coordinated care, I believe that choosing a good surgical team is essential to getting the best cosmetic result.

Some surgeons argue that it is "safer" to wait until after the mastectomy is performed before reconstruction should be considered. It is hard to understand this position unless the surgeon is thinking of his or her own scheduling issues. There is no evidence that waiting for reconstruction is safer. Most women will have a much better result from reconstruction when it is done at the same time as mastectomy because the tissues have not been sacrificed to close the wound and have not scarred down to the chest wall. If you are interested in reconstruction, you may have to insist on seeing a plastic surgeon before your mastectomy.

• Ask yourself whether you truly feel comfortable with the doctor. If you do not feel a personal trust for the doctor taking care of you, perhaps you should talk to other doctors before you make a final decision.

• Finally, make sure the surgeon is board-certified, trained, and experienced in the procedure you are considering. Typically, patients are not referred to a plastic surgeon if the surgeon has not previously demonstrated competence with breast reconstruction.

Breast reconstruction is an important part of treatment for breast cancer and should never be discounted as merely cosmetic. Each choice for reconstruction will provide you with a different result, and each has its own risks and costs. Only by understanding the choices and their likely outcomes can you fully consider your needs and determine which choice is right for you.

Weighing the Choices

Type of operation:	Tissue expander followed by implant	Latissimus flap with implant	TRAM flap
Implant risk of leakage	Some risk	Some risk	No risk
Implant risk of "hard" scar (First five years)	30 to 40%	30 to 40%	No risk
Need for future procedures	Common	Less common	Rare
Length of surgery (Approximate)	One hour	Three hours	Six hours
Hospital stay	One to two days	Two to three days	Four to Five days
Abdominal wall pain	None	None	Significant for two to six weeks
Healing of back wound	None	Two to three weeks	None
Natural result	Good (50 to 60 percent)	Better (70 to 85 percent)	Best (90 to 99 percent)
Effect of radiation therapy on result	Poor	Poor if implant used	Radiation well-tolerated if transferred as free flap
Surgical fees (Varies by plastic surgeon)	$3,000	$5,000	$8,000

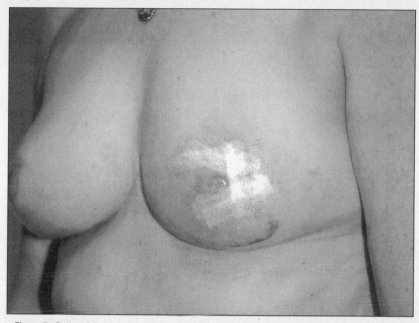

Figure 7. Patient following biopsy with wound tapes in place and some bruising evident.

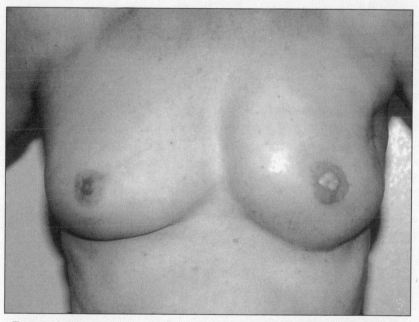

Figure 8. A tissue expander has been removed and replaced with a saline-filled "permanent" implant. After patients are happy with the location and size of the implant, the nipple/areolar complex can be reconstructed.

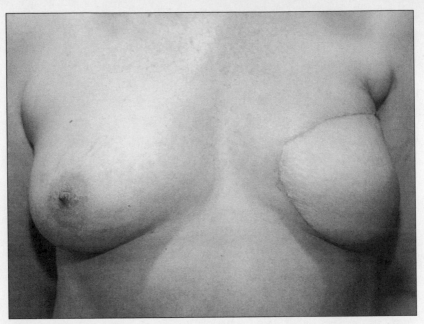

Figure 9. A patient with a previous history of radiation therapy developed a recurrence of cancer in her breast skin necessitating removal of the skin with the underlying breast tissue. A TRAM flap has been brought up to fill the defect created by the removal of the breast and a significant amount of breast skin.

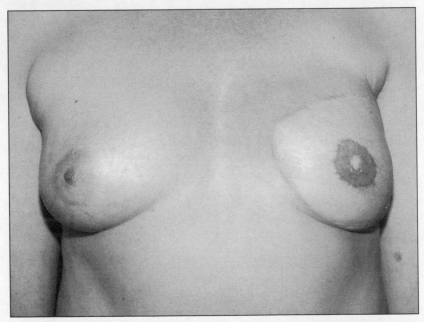

Figure 10. The nipple/areolar complex has been reconstructed. The breast reconstruction is soft and natural to the touch. The patient's original breast skin could not be preserved in this case because it had been irradiated prior to mastectomy.

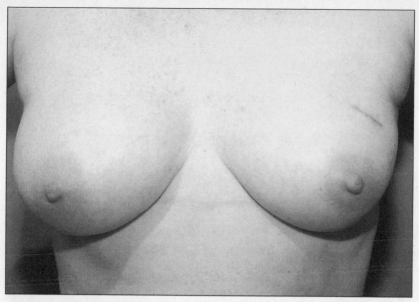

Figure 11. This patient has been diagnosed with breast cancer using an open technique. The resulting scar will be removed during mastectomy.

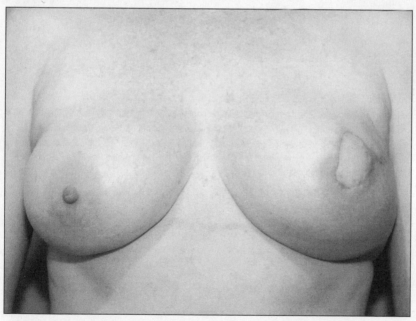

Figure 12. Almost all of the breast skin has been preserved, including the areolar tissue. The nipple has been taken with the breast gland. A TRAM flap has been brought up and placed in the skin envelope. This photograph was taken two months after the mastectomy was done and the flap transferred to the chest wall.

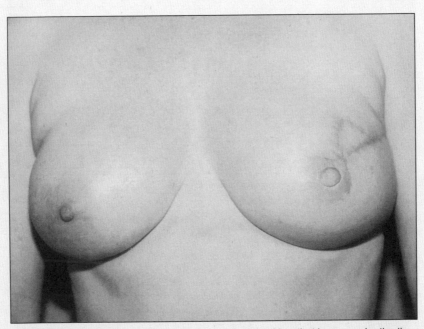

Figure 13. A nipple/areolar complex has been reconstructed in this patient by reapproximating the saved areolar skin around a newly constructed nipple. Pigment can be added to the nipple using tattoo techniques. To an observer, this reconstructed breast feels the same as the patient's opposite breast. To the patient, the sensation of the saved skin feels like her opposite breast, but nipple sensation is obviously absent.

CHAPTER TEN

Chemotherapy, Hormone Therapy, and the Stages of Breast Cancer

By Alexander C. Black, M.D.

Breast cancer treatment can be thought of as two separate, but related issues: local treatment for the breast (surgery and radiation) and systemic therapy. Chemotherapy and hormone therapy are generally referred to as *adjuvant* (additional) or *systemic therapy* because these treatments work through the bloodstream to affect the entire body to treat possible microscopic or metastatic disease. Treatment may be used to potentially cure, or to control side effects of the disease (palliate), and perhaps to prolong survival. Not every woman receives the same treatment regimen, because cancer has tremendous biologic variability. The type of cancer you have, the stage to which the disease has progressed, and the cancer's characteristics will all affect prognosis (or likely outcome) and your treatment plan.

Some women with early stage breast cancer may be treated with chemotherapy and/or hormone therapy. Although chemotherapy is typically given after surgery, it is sometimes used preoperatively to treat a large aggressive cancer and, in general, it is given before radiation. Certain chemotherapy drugs, such as doxorubicin or methotrexate, should not be given at the same time as radiation therapy, because they can enhance the toxicities of radiation. A chemotherapy regimen called

CMF (which stands for the chemotherapy drugs cyclophosphamide, methotrexate, and 5 flourouracil) can be given during radiation therapy, if the drug methotrexate is deleted during that time.

Has Your Cancer Spread?

To determine the best course of treatment for your cancer, your doctor will try to understand whether and to what extent the cancer may have spread, or metastasized, outside the breast to distant parts of the body through the lymph ducts or bloodstream. It is difficult to assess how far any cancer has spread, but doctors can make their best guess with the available diagnostic tools. If it appears that your cancer is confined to the breast, one path of treatment is indicated and, if it seems that the cancer has spread, treatment will follow another direction.

The first step in determining whether cancer has spread is called *clinical staging*. In any possible stage of breast cancer, you should have, at minimum, a detailed medical history taken; a physical exam; breast-imaging studies, like mammography; a chest X ray to see if the cancer has traveled to the lungs; and screening chemistries with liver function tests to look for evidence of the spread of cancer to the liver.

If the initial clinical evaluation suggests that the cancer may have spread, you should then receive additional tests, such as a bone scan to see if cancer has spread to the bone, and a CT scan (CT stands for computerized tomography, a computer controlled X ray system that can take cross-sectional images of a part of the body) to rule out spread to visceral organs, such as the lung, liver, and brain. A PET scan (or positron emission tomography), which is used to identify abnormal areas of metabolism in the body associated with the presence of cancer, is currently being explored as another way of staging breast cancer.

If the cancer appears to be localized to the breast, the next step is usually surgery. The pathologist's analysis of the surgical specimen, which includes the cancer and lymph nodes, is critical to determining your risk of recurrence of cancer and to determining the best way to treat your cancer. From a medical oncologist's perspective, the three most important cancer characteristics of the TNM system are:

• **T**, or the size the tumor.

• **N**, the number of axillary (or armpit) nodes involved with the tumor. The presence of cancer in the lymph nodes suggests whether the cancer has spread.

• **M**, the evidence of metastases, or cancer spread outside the breast.

Estrogen and Progesterone Hormone Receptors (ER and PR)

In addition to understanding the TNM system, it's important to know whether your tumor has cells with estrogen and/or progesterone receptors. Estrogen and progesterone are naturally occurring female hormones that can stimulate the growth of certain tumors comprised of cells with receptors for estrogen and progesterone. Estrogen and progesterone can bind to these receptors and promote cell division. Hormone manipulation therapies like tamoxifen can interact with the same receptors to block the action of estrogen and kill ER/PR positive cells. Your ER/PR status will determine whether your cancer will respond to hormone manipulation therapy.

The Stages of Cancer

We use the TNM system to stage cancer. There are four primary stages of cancer, classified as stages I through IV. Whatever your staging work-up shows, there are therapies available to improve your quality of life and prolong survival. Stages I through III are potentially curable, but Stage IV, or widespread disease, is not.

• **Stage I** represents a small tumor, or a tumor equal to or less than two centimeters in diameter (denoted as T1) with no lymph node involvement (N0). Stages I through III are potentially curable, although the risk of relapse, despite aggressive anti-cancer therapy increases with each stage.

• **Stage II** represents either a larger tumor (greater than two centimeters and up to five centimeters) and/or a cancer that has spread to lymph nodes unattached to each other or to tissue (called *nonfixed nodes*) (N1) or a very large tumor (over 5 centimeters) without any lymph node involvement.

• **Stage III** can describe a combination of any of the four following situations: cancer in lymph nodes that are fixed to each other or to nearby tissue (fixed axillary lymph node metastases, or N2); cancer spread to the lymph nodes beneath the breast next to the sternum (internal mammary lymph node metastases, N3); a very large tumor (T3) with involvement of either fixed or nonfixed lymph nodes (N1 or N2); or cancer that has invaded the chest wall or skin (T4).

• **Stage IV** means that the cancer has spread outside the breast and nearby lymph nodes, or distant metastases. The median survival time for people with Stage IV cancer is three years, but this is based on a statistical average and cannot necessarily be applied to any one individual. Some people with Stage IV cancer survive over ten years. Rarely, people with Stage IV cancer survive without anti-cancer treatment, a fact that underscores the tremendous differences in the biology of cancer and its behavior in the body.

Other Factors That Affect Treatment Decisions and Prognosis

Decisions about the risk of relapse and the best treatment choices for your cancer are based on a number of factors including the TNM system (tumor, nodes, metastases) above and other characteristics of your cancer such as:

• **Histology.** Most cancers that occur in the breast are adenocarcinomas or cancers that occur in the glandular tissues. There is a great variation in the way that these cancer cells appear under the microscope. They are of different types and structures, with some forms being less aggressive than others. The type of cancer you have can affect your prognosis. For example, tubular (tubelike), mucinous (mucus-producing), and papillary cancers are forms of breast cancer that are less aggressive and confer a better outlook. However, cell structure is most important to prognosis in early stage disease.

• **Her2/neu** is another important factor in prognosis and treatment for metastatic and potentially for early stage breast cancer. In some people, breast cells may overproduce a gene related to a growth factor receptor called her2/neu, which tells the cell to divide faster. The overexpression of her2/neu is associated with a more aggressive form of cancer. Yet, a specially designed antibody called *Herceptin* has been shown to be effective in targeting cells that make too much of this growth factor receptor. Antibodies are proteins made by the immune system that recognize and fight foreign substances in the body. Recent studies suggest that Herceptin recognizes and binds to the her2/neu protein on the surface of the cell and sends a signal through the her2/neu receptor that induces cancer cells to die. This therapy appears to have a synergistic, or more than additive, effect when used with certain chemotherapy drugs, like paclitaxel, and it is an exciting example of the advances being made in cancer research.

• Other characteristics of cell DNA, like **percent S phase,** which tells us how rapidly cells are dividing, and **ploidy,** which refers to the number of chromosome sets in a cell and can indicate whether a cell has an abnormal number of chromosomes, may affect prognosis but do no yet affect treatment recommendations. Some European studies suggest a role for bone marrow aspiration and biopsy with special tissue stains to look for breast cancer. The presence of cancer cells in bone marrow may suggest a poorer prognosis, much as involvement with the lymph nodes does. This procedure is not yet standard, however, for evaluating early stage breast cancer in the United States.

Chemotherapy and Hormone Therapy: Systemic Treatment

Even in the early stages of cancer, cells can travel from the primary site through the blood and lymph systems to other parts of the body. Chemotherapy consists of medications given to kill these cells and to keep cancer from spreading and recurring. Adjuvant therapy may prevent a relapse, which in turn might cure someone who might otherwise not be cured.

Although chemotherapy has toxic effects on normal cells and tissues, the drugs are more toxic to cancer cells. Given the explosion of information on the molecular and genetic mechanisms of disease, we have both a better understanding of how chemotherapy drugs preferentially treat cancer cells and what cell characteristics make them a promising target for new anti-cancer therapies. The last decade has seen the development of several drugs with impressive activity in breast cancer, including paclitaxel, docetaxel, capecitabine, vinorelbine, and gemcitabine. Not every woman with breast cancer will be treated with chemotherapy. The decision to treat your cancer with chemotherapy and the type of chemotherapy drugs used in your treatment will be based on all of the information your doctor has about your disease after the pathological assessment. Certain characteristics of your cancer may influence what type of chemotherapy is used. For example, if you have ER/PR positive tumors, the addition of paclitaxel to doxorubicin (Adriamycin) may provide you with little benefit. Likewise, women with tumors that overexpress her2/neu may get more benefit from doxorubicin.

It's safe to say that chemotherapy may be the most dreaded aspect of cancer treatment as most people have heard stories about its horrible side effects. A variety of new drugs as well as a conscious new effort by clinical researchers to carefully measure the quality of life of patients undergoing cancer treatments have made side effects much less likely.

Administering Chemotherapy

Chemotherapy drugs are usually administered intravenously, through an IV, usually in a vein of the forearm. It is virtually always given in an outpatient setting by a trained oncology nurse, who should be certified. Generally, you will first be given an antinausea drug orally or through an IV before chemotherapy.

The need for repeated IV administration of chemotherapy and the risk of severe injury if certain drugs like doxorubicin (Adriamycin) leak out of a vein often make durable IV access desirable. Durable IV access

GETTING A SECOND OPINION ABOUT CHEMOTHERAPY

Getting a second medical opinion is always reasonable and shouldn't disturb those involved in your treatment. If you are receiving treatment in a community hospital and there is an academic center nearby—for example, a university hospital—you might contact a medical oncologist in that setting for additional academic perspective.

refers to an intravenous device that can remain in place for at least several weeks and up to many months. Subcutaneous port devices, or devices implanted under the skin, including the Port-A-Cath brand catheter, can be placed surgically. Blood samples can be drawn and chemotherapy can be administered by sticking an appropriately sized needle through the skin overlying the device and through the outer membrane of the device. The subcutaneous devices are less likely to become infected and require less maintenance than IV access that involves tubing that is partly outside the skin, such as a PICC line. A Port-A-Cath is a quarter-sized membrane placed under the skin in the upper chest.

The surgeon will place the Port-A-Cath. The Port-A-Cath is attached to a small tube that is typically inserted into a major vein located in the chest called the subclavian vein, although other veins can be used. The operation is done under local anesthetic and takes about 45 minutes to perform. You will have a small scar where the Port-A-Cath is inserted and a small scar where the incision was made to find the vein.

I chose the Port-A-Cath and went through an outpatient surgery to implant it into my chest. The procedure was easy. The device gave me the look of an alien with a round nipple protruding under the skin of my upper chest. It was one of the best decisions I made and became a badge of courage that I was proud to show off. • Dianne

A Port-A-Cath is difficult, but well worth doing. I had one in my chest and one in my arm. I found the one in my arm a little easier to deal with. I didn't cover it. I wore short-sleeved-shirts. It just sits in a little crook in the arm. It wasn't as in the way as the one in my chest. • Joelle

I was more scared of the Port-A-Cath than chemo. I didn't want one, but it makes treatment easier, because there's one needle, and that's it.
• Cynthia

With any long-term IV, there is risk of a catheter infection that could potentially spread to the blood and the risk of a clot forming around the catheter and clogging the vein. Catheter infections require treatment with antibiotics; catheter-related clots call for treatment with blood thinners like heparin and coumadin. Generally speaking, these are unusual complications. Recent studies have shown that a low-dose treatment of blood-thinning therapy with coumadin can significantly reduce the risk of clot formation with minimal risk of significant bleeding. Almost all standard chemotherapy treatments are required for more than one or two months, thus a Port-A-Cath is typically the most desirable means of administration because of the lower risk of infection and greater convenience to the woman being treated.

Timing and Duration of Chemotherapy

Chemotherapy can be given within a few weeks of surgery, because wound healing is not substantially affected. The duration of your chemotherapy treatment can vary from a minimum of three months to a maximum of nine months. As mentioned previously, radiation therapy is generally given after chemotherapy. Radiation oncologists prefer to give radiation therapy within six months after surgery to decrease the risk of recurrence of cancer in the breast area. Although chemotherapy helps decrease the risk of local recurrence somewhat, surgery and radiation therapy are much more important to eliminating recurrence of the cancer in the breast overall.

I was more petrified of chemotherapy than anything I had gone through, because it was so unknown. I had heard horror stories, but it wasn't as

bad as I thought it would be. My white blood counts went down, and I had to take Neupogen. My oncology nurse, who was wonderful, taught me how to give myself a shot, and I thought I was going to be okay. But I just sat there for an hour looking at the needle. Finally, my husband's dad, who I call my father-in-love, said he would do it for me. · Linda L.

I felt very sick during chemotherapy. I had some hair loss but not all. I continued working, and the people at work served as a wonderful support for me. They made me laugh. · Linda R.

Side Effects of Chemotherapy

Because chemotherapy can injure normal rapidly dividing tissues like hair follicles, mouth- and gut-lining cells, as well as bone marrow cells, which produce white and red blood cells and platelets, you may experience unpleasant side effects. Mild hair thinning to complete hair loss caused by injury to the hair follicles can be very difficult for many women. Nausea and vomiting are induced by the effect of chemotherapy on the lining of your stomach and on the vomit control centers in the brainstem. You may also experience mouth sores and changes in your appetite or bowel habits. Less commonly, certain

> Chemotherapy is not what it once was. Over the last 15 years, new chemotherapy drugs and new supportive measures have been introduced that lessen side effects and have made chemotherapy both easier to tolerate and more effective, even with very aggressive chemotherapy regimens.

drugs cause organ-specific complications. Adriamycin (doxorubicin) can hurt heart muscles, although not in low doses. Taxanes, like Taxol or Taxotere, which we will talk about in this chapter, can cause aching of the muscles and joints and neurotoxicity, or tingling in the fingers and toes, numbness, and unusual sensitivity of the skin. Some chemotherapy drugs have more side effects than others. With doxorubicin (Adriamycin), hair loss is complete and fatigue and nausea may be more pronounced. However, with supportive treatments to ease side effects, most women can tolerate even the most serious side effects. Talk to your medical oncologist about possible side effects and treatments to ameliorate them.

I made the decision to go shopping for wigs before I needed one. I bought one to look exactly like me and another to be a blond for the first time. My hairdresser cut and styled both to look very much like my real hair. I felt ready to enter this new territory. • Dianne

You lose your hair with Adriamycin. I found out that I have a very round head with no bumps or dents. I didn't find wigs to be comfortable so I wore hats. Some evenings I'd go out to Hollywood and fit right in just going bald. Once my hair started growing, the hats were gone. We'd take my daughter to the drugstore to pick out hair dye, and she'd dye my hair all sorts of colors while I had a crew cut. • Joelle

Nobody told me I was going to lose my hair. On Friday the 13th, as I was combing my hair, half of it just fell out. It was a big matted rat of hair,

CHOOSING YOUR MEDICAL ONCOLOGIST

When you have a choice of practitioners, make sure to ask your medical oncologist:

- Are you board-certified?

- Are you affiliated with a medical center where I might be able to find out about investigational therapies and the latest in treatment options?

Ask yourself:

- Does the medical oncologist help you understand the risks and benefits of your treatment options?

- Do you feel comfortable with the office where you will receive treatment, often called an infusion center?

- Are you comfortable with the oncology nurse? Does she or he explain the treatment process to you?

- How do the front office staff members treat you? Are they courteous? Do they answer your questions?

For more information, see Chapter 19, "How to Get the Best Care and Treatment."

which we now have hanging in the garage with a sign over it that reads "roadkill" because that's exactly what it looked like. · Cynthia

We were at a softball game sitting on the bleachers. All of the sudden, a wind just came up and my hat with hair attached went flying. I wasn't sure what to do as I sat there with my bald little head. I thought for sure I'd make a scene chasing this "thing" with my naked head. All my friend could think to do was to empty her purse on my head. It was kind of funny but also very embarrassing. I'm glad that's over with. · Linda L.

Chemotherapy can accelerate the tendency toward menopause and may tip perimenopausal women into menopause, causing symptoms of menopause in some women. But it's important to note that women often can and do get pregnant after adjuvant therapy. There is no convincing reproducible data that have shown that pregnancy decreases breast cancer survival. Of course, each woman must discuss plans for pregnancy in-depth with her medical treatment team.

Injury to the bone marrow causes suppression of blood counts, which can increase your risk of infection from low white blood cell counts, anemia due to low red blood cell counts, and bleeding from low platelets. These are among the most difficult side effects, but fortunately there are a number of interventions to ameliorate these complications.

New Drugs Can Control Side Effects of Chemotherapy

The growth of chemotherapeutic and biologic treatment options has been complemented by dramatic improvements in the control of symptoms caused by chemotherapy. A whole new class of drugs that work on the serotonin pathways to control nausea, called *anti-emetics*, like ondansetron, granisetron, and dolasetron, have substantially reduced nausea and vomiting even in the most aggressive chemotherapy regimens. Special hormones that stimulate blood cell growth, called *hematopoietic cytokines*, have reduced the degree and duration of suppression of blood cell counts after chemotherapy. White blood cells grow back faster with filgrastim (Neupogen) and sargramostim (Leukine), both of which have been shown to reduce the occurrence of fevers requiring hospitalization. Erythropoietin (Procrit or Epogen) stimulates red blood cells and has been shown to improve anemia and reduce transfusion requirements in people receiving chemotherapy that causes blood count suppression. Interleukin 2 (Neumega), thrombopoietin, or megakaryocyte growth development factor (MGDF) stimulate recovery of platelets to help to prevent spontaneous bleeding.

Chemotherapy can cause menopausal symptoms, particularly hot flashes. Because standard estrogen supplements seem to increase the risk of a recurrence of breast cancer, a series of nonhormonal treatments have been studied and appear to be active in reducing symptoms. These therapies include low-dose clonidine (Catapres), which is an antihypertensive, and low-dose antidepressants, particularly Effexor, and a low-dose progestational agent like Megace. Dr. Cohen addresses other strategies to reduce some of the difficulties created by menopausal symptoms in Chapter 15, "The Estrogen Dilemma and Breast Cancer."

Talk to your doctor about your fears and your needs. Be proactive. I needed sleep medication. I needed antinausea medication. If a drug is not working for you, tell the doctors. Do what you can to get through chemotherapy. There are many drugs worth purchasing or finding. If your insurance doesn't cover them, perhaps your doctor can give you free samples. • Joelle

Controlling Pain

Pain can be a part of breast cancer and its treatment, but the goal is to control and minimize pain as much as possible. The source of pain may be surgery or radiation, or it can arise as a side effect of a medication or from the swelling of an organ. A tumor that is close to the sensory nerves and invades into or presses upon the nerves can cause pain.

When breast cancer spreads, it most commonly spreads to the bone, thus improvement in pain control intervention and therapies to prevent bone complications has had a substantial impact on cancer care. Studies have produced very effective graduated methods for delivering pain control that involve treatments ranging from nonsteroidal anti-inflammatory drugs (like ibuprofen), neuroleptics, antidepressants, which have pain-relieving properties, and weak to strong narcotics. Generally, your physician will begin with the weakest medication with the fewest side effects and may gradually move to stronger medications. Narcotics are available in long- and short-acting formulations as well as oral, injection, or topical form. Other invasive strategies for pain control include nerve blocks (intravenous or spinal injections) and continuous infusion pumps. An infusion pump is another way to infuse pain medication quickly. This is an external device that looks like a Walkman with a shoulder strap with a tube that connects to a PICC line or Port-A-Cath to infuse the pain medication.

> ### BISPHOSPHONATES SLOW THE PROGRESSION OF CANCER TO THE BONE
>
> Bisphosphonates, like pamidronate, are drugs developed to help lower high blood calcium levels. They have been shown to slow the progression of cancer spread to the bone and decrease the occurrence of fractures in people with breast cancer that involves the bone. Although both oral and intravenous bisphosphonates are available, pamidronate is the best-studied agent and remains the standard, given every three to four weeks.

Tamoxifen and Other Hormone Manipulation Therapies

It's been known for decades that estrogen and progesterone, female hormones normally occurring in the body and produced primarily by the ovaries, can stimulate certain breast cancer tumors, those that are positive for estrogen or progesterone receptors. In the past, estrogen production was hindered by the removal of the ovaries; today, however, there are a number of well-tolerated oral and injection treatments to inhibit hormone production.

Tamoxifen (Nolvadex) is the best-studied and current front-line treatment in both early and metastatic breast cancer. Taken in pill form daily, tamoxifen is what's known as a *selective estrogen receptor modulator (SERM)*; it acts as an antiestrogen, blocking the estrogen receptor on the surface of the cell and, by other less-understood mechanisms, killing cancer cells that are estrogen and/or progesterone (ER/PR) positive. (If a tumor expresses the progesterone receptor, it means that the cancer is still receptive to estrogen and is an indication for tamoxifen.) While tamoxifen acts as an antiestrogen attacking breast cancer and promoting hot flashes and vaginal dryness, it also acts as a pro-estrogen, stimulating the growth of the lining of the uterus, inhibiting osteoporosis, and improving your cholesterol profile. There are other side effects from tamoxifen:

• In addition to hot flashes, tamoxifen increases the risk of endometrial, or uterine, cancer from approximately one in a thousand women over a five-year period of time to approximately three in a thousand over five years of continuous use of tamoxifen.

• As with natural menopause, premature menopause induced by chemotherapy and/or tamoxifen may be associated with mood swings and depression. There is also a controversial association with subtle memory loss or reduction in mental acuity.

• In women over 50, there is a two- to threefold increase in the risk of deep vein clots in the thigh or pelvis and of clots that can travel to the lung, called *pulmonary emboli.*

• There may be a slight increased risk of cataracts, weight gain, rare blood count disorders, or allergic reactions.

While there are risks, tamoxifen is generally known to be so safe that it has been studied as a preventative treatment in women without breast cancer but at high risk for the disease. A large randomized study, known as the *P1 Trial*, confirmed about a 50-percent reduction in the development of breast cancer over five years in high-risk women on tamoxifen. The efficacy of tamoxifen was suggested previously by the decreased incidences of breast cancer in the opposite breast when taken by women for a prior diagnosed breast cancer. Because women taking raloxifene (Evista) saw a similar benefit in an osteoporosis prevention trial, a large, randomized clinical trial called the STAR trial, is currently under way to compare raloxifene with tamoxifen for breast cancer prevention and side effects, particularly with respect to the reduction of endometrial cancer risk. Women at higher risk for breast cancer based on age greater than 60, multiple breast biopsies, higher risk benign breast biopsy results, and a first-degree relative with a history of breast cancer are eligible to participate.

Women with BRCA-1 and BRCA-2 mutations (see below) are clearly at high risk for breast cancer, yet it's not clear what role tamoxifen has versus bilateral mastectomy (removing both breasts) and possible removal of the ovaries (oopherectomy) in the prevention of breast cancer in women with BRCA-1 or BRCA-2 mutation. Recent studies have shown that preventative (prophylactic) bilateral mastectomies reduce the risk of breast cancer by about 90 percent in women at high risk.

Screening for BRCA-1 and 2

Studies of families with an extremely high occurrence of breast cancer led to the identification of the culprit: mutated, or damaged, genes BRCA-1 and 2. However, mutations in these genes are responsible for only a small minority of breast cancers and are also associated with an increased risk of other cancers, particularly ovarian cancers with BRCA-1 mutations.

Screening for these mutations should be considered when:

- You have a family history of several breast cancers or breast and ovarian cancer in first-degree relatives, such as a mother, sister, or daughter.

- You have breast cancer and are under 30 years of age.

There are disadvantages to screening:

- The genetic sequencing required to test for BRCA-1 and 2 mutations is laborious, time-consuming, and expensive.

- Many insurance plans will not cover the cost of several thousand dollars, even if a mutation is identified.

- Some women with identified genetic mutations may feel compelled to take drastic preventative measures like the surgical removal of the breasts or ovaries.

• In addition, patients may have more difficulty obtaining or paying for medical, disability, and life insurance.

Other Hormonal Treatments for Metastatic Disease

There are a variety of well-tolerated hormonal treatments for metastatic breast cancer. Therapies like tamoxifen and toremifene act as anti-estrogens, blocking the action of estrogen. There are several other new antiestrogens in development. Additional methods of suppressing estrogen production include removal of the ovaries (which is seldom done because of newer therapies), radiation, and more recently by the use of a new class of drugs called *LHRH agonists* (luteinizing hormone releasing hormone-agonists), like leuprolide or goserelin, which can be injected under the skin and which suppress the production of estrogen by the ovaries. Luteinizing hormones are pituitary hormones that play an important role in ovulation. Another new class of drugs called *aro-*

STEM CELL TRANSPLANTS AND HIGH-DOSE CHEMOTHERAPY

Over the last decade, there have been a number of studies to determine the role of high-dose chemotherapy in the treatment of metastatic breast cancer or people at high risk of relapse, including women with Stage II breast cancer and ten or more positive lymph nodes. Peripheral blood stem-cell transplants (PBSCT) involve the collection of young blood cells capable of maturing into red and white cells and platelets that circulate normally in the bloodstream. These are the stem cells. After chemotherapy and cytokine treatment (generally, Neupogen, which stimulates blood cell growth), the blood cells were collected by a special blood-filtering procedure known as *apheresis*. The patient was then treated with high-dose chemotherapy after which she was reinfused with her harvested blood cells, allowing for a more rapid recovery of white and red blood cells and platelets. Although initial results appeared promising, the vast majority of larger studies have not shown a clear advantage of this treatment. But studies continue to explore the possibility that different high-dose chemotherapy drugs or different combinations of standard- and high-dose chemotherapy drugs might prove superior to the best standard chemotherapy alone.

matase inhibitors work to stop synthesis of estrogen from the ovaries and adrenal glands and appear to be at least as effective as tamoxifen. These include the nonsteroidal inhibitors, anastrozol and letrozole, and the steroidal inhibitors, formestane and exemestane.

Studies have confirmed the relative equivalence of antiestrogen treatments, LHRH agonists, and aromatase inhibitors in the treatment of metastases as well as the superiority of antiestrogens and aromastasc inhibitors over progestational agents, such as megestrol acetate. Androgen therapies, like halotestin, are rarely used today because other drugs have been found to be more effective and do not cause masculinization like facial hair growth or a deeper voice. If you have ER/PR positive metastatic cancer, you may choose to undergo a series of different hormonal treatments, as cancer with these characteristics often responds to several hormonal agents in sequence. Recent studies suggest that initial therapy with aromatase inhibitors may lead to a more superior outcome than initial therapy with tamoxifen.

Adjuvant Treatment's Various Stages

DCIS, or ductal carcinoma in situ.

Since the advent of routine screening mammography, many women are diagnosed with carcinoma in situ. Carcinoma in situ is a collection of cancer cells that usually cannot be felt and have not yet invaded or violated tissue boundaries (that is, they are still trapped in the ducts that carry milk) but represent a high potential for invasive breast cancer, if not surgically removed, in the future. As with invasive breast cancer, treatment of ductal CIS has been determined through clinical trials. Ductal CIS, or DCIS, occurs in the milk ducts and is treated like early stage breast cancer requiring surgery, usually followed by radiation therapy. If untreated, there is a risk that DCIS could become invasive. Because DCIS is a marker for increased risk of breast cancer, you may decide to take tamoxifen for five years, which has been shown to reduce the risk of breast cancer by 50 percent.

Lobular CIS, or LCIS, which is confined to the lobules where milk is produced in the breast, is also a pre-cancer. Like DCIS, LCIS increases the lifetime risk of breast cancer, but to a lesser degree. It is not treated with surgery or radiation but provides a rationale for preventative treatment with tamoxifen.

Stages I and II

Stages I and II represent early stage cancer when cure is the goal. Typically, women with Stage I and II diagnoses will have surgery to remove the tumor and sample the lymph nodes. After surgery, the findings from your breast surgery and lymph node removal will be assessed to help your medical oncologist determine whether chemotherapy and/or hormone therapy will be right for you. If your overall health is good and you have a cancer of a centimeter or more, systemic therapy is generally recommended. In cases with a favorable histology (such as pure tubular, mucinous, or papillary tumors), adjuvant (additional) therapy is generally recommended in tumors greater than or equal to three centimeters.

Tamoxifen taken at 20 milligrams daily for five years following radiation therapy is standard treatment for women whose tumors were ER/IR positive. The more complicated and debatable issue is whether chemotherapy will be a part of treatment, particularly if you will also receive tamoxifen. Tamoxifen reduces the risk of recurrence of breast cancer in patients with hormone receptor positive tumors by about 30 percent, similar to that reduction in risk with chemotherapy alone. Standard chemotherapy appears to reduce relapse by an additional 5 percent. Preliminary studies suggest that for people with axillary lymph node involvement, the addition of a taxane, like paclitaxel, to other chemotherapy drugs like doxorubicin (Adriamycin) and cyclophosfamide (Cytoxan) appears to reduce the rate of relapse by 50 percent.

The absolute benefit to you in the reduction of your risk for a relapse depends on the risk of relapse after local therapy, which, as you know, means surgery with or without radiation. We measure the risk of relapse based on all the information we have about your cancer from staging the disease, including the size of your tumor, the number of lymph nodes involved, whether the cancer has spread, whether the tumor is ER/PR positive, as well as other characteristics of cancer discussed above. The risk of relapse increases dramatically with the number of lymph nodes involved from about 15 percent with a small tumor (less than two centimeters) and no lymph node involvement to greater than 80 percent with ten or more lymph nodes involved.

If you are over 80, when the risk of dying from other causes becomes a real possibility, you and your doctor may want to have candid discussions about the benefit of chemotherapy to you under these circumstances. Every patient should have frank discussions with her medical oncologist about the risks and benefits of adjuvant therapies in the context of her personal goals and values.

Stage III

Because Stage III cancer can have a combination of features, there is no defined treatment for this stage. Some women with large breast cancers that are not involved with the skin or the chest wall and do not have fixed lymph node involvement can be treated like women with Stage II cancer. Generally, this means surgery, followed by chemotherapy and radiation therapy. Women whose cancers are very large and that show other unfavorable characteristics are treated with aggressive chemotherapy before surgery, called *neoadjuvant therapy*. Although treatment with chemotherapy before surgery does not affect survival rates, a tumor that shrinks with preoperative chemotherapy proves the cancer's responsiveness to chemotherapy. As discussed in Chapter 6, "Saving the Breast," preoperative chemotherapy can occasionally prevent mastectomy if the cancer has shrunk enough to allow for breast-saving surgery. It should be stated, however, that the best form of preoperative chemotherapy has not been defined, and the role of chemotherapy after surgery in people who have also received chemotherapy before surgery remains undefined. Before embarking on this type of treatment, the possibility of the cancer continuing to grow during chemotherapy must be considered and the risks must be carefully weighed.

Stage IV

Generally, the main objective in Stage IV cancer is to prolong survival and improve overall quality of life. Fortunately, many studies have shown that both chemotherapy and/or hormone therapy can accomplish those goals, avoiding or delaying serious effects of the disease, including pain.

There are several established guidelines for treatment. If you have ER/PR positive breast cancer and a slowly progressing disease confined to the soft tissues and/or bone, you can be treated with sequential hormone therapy until the disease has progressed on three or four different treatments. Chemotherapy drugs in combination result in a higher response rate or tumor shrinkage than the use of a single chemotherapy drug, but has not been shown to increase survival when compared to the use of chemotherapy drugs in sequence—that is, given one after the other. A family of drugs called the *anthracyclines*, like doxorubicin (Adriamycin) and epirubicin (Ellence); and taxanes, like paclitaxel (Taxol) and docetaxel (Taxotere), are the most effective chemotherapy drugs in breast cancer. An oral form of the chemotherapy drug 5 fluorouracil, capecitabine (Xeloda), is one of the latest additions to chemotherapy treatment and seems to be well-tolerated and effective. Over the last decade, several other chemotherapy drugs that are active in breast cancer have been developed, including gemcitabine (Gemzar) and vinorelbine (Navelbine). Stem cell transplants, which we talked about earlier, don't seem to improve survival rate compared to the best chemotherapy.

Supportive care to relieve symptoms may be the best answer if your disease has progressed on three different chemotherapy regimens:

• Surgery and radiation can be used to ease symptoms of metastatic breast cancer. Surgery can be used to stabilize bone fractures or control spinal cord compression, if it is progressing or recurring despite radiation. Sometimes a woman who has experienced an isolated metastasis after a long disease-free period can have the area removed surgically, particularly in the brain.

• Radiation is very effective in controlling metastases to the bone-causing pain or potential fractures and to the brain when neurological complications exist or are threatened. Radiation can also be very helpful in controlling soft tissue metastases, for example, if you experience a recurrence in the chest wall after mastectomy.

• As mentioned in the section on supportive care, a drug called *pamidronate*, given intravenously, can retard the progress of the spread to the bone.

• Surgeons can help control pain a great deal by performing nerve blocks or placing permanent intravenous pain control devices, like Port-A-Caths or infusion pumps.

What Are the Risk Factors?

There are a host of risk factors associated with breast cancer. A personal or family history is most important. The more first-degree relatives, such as a mother, sister, or daughter, or second-degree relatives, such as an aunt or grandmother, who had breast cancer, and the earlier the age at which they developed breast cancer, the more likely you are to develop breast cancer. The occurrence of bilateral breast cancer, or cancer in both breasts, in a family member also increases risk. A small proportion of women with a family history of breast cancer have one of several breast cancer syndromes, including breast-ovarian cancer syndromes (which we'll talk about in a moment), Li-Fraumeni, Cowden's disease, or Muir-Torre syndromes. These latter three conditions are particularly rare.

WHAT IS BREAST CANCER AND WHAT CAUSES IT?

Breast cancer is the most common form of cancer among women and the second most common cause of cancer deaths after lung cancer. Breast cancer occurs when normal breast cells suffer damage to their genetic material, or DNA (deoxyribonucleic acid). The breast cells that turn cancerous are generally from glandular tissues, and are called *adenocarcinomas*. *Adeno* literally means gland. (Other types of cancer, such as lymphoma, cancer that begins in the lymph nodes, and sarcomas, which are cancers that begin in the muscle cells, occur in the breast, but they are much less common.) If a breast glandular cell survives the initial genetic injury and is able to reproduce, or divide, the daughter cells with that initial mutation can potentially suffer further genetic injuries. Current thinking suggests that several different cancer-predisposing injuries, or mutations, must occur within in a cell before that cell becomes malignant. Once a cell has become malignant, or cancerous, it must divide many times before a clinically significant, recognizable cancer develops. A one-centimeter-in-diameter (less-than-a-half-inch) cancer represents one billion cancer cells. Hence, the process of cell transformation and cancer growth is thought to happen over years.

One of the most exciting developments in breast cancer research over the last decade has been the improvement in understanding of the genetic changes associated with breast cancer development. This can be shown by the identification of inherited mutations of specific genes associated with breast cancer syndromes. Cowden's disease is characterized by mutations in the PTEN gene and by multiple hamartomas, or benign blood vessel tumors, that involve the breast, thyroid gland, skin, and brain. People with Cowden's disease have an increased risk of breast and thyroid cancers. Li-Fraumeni syndrome is caused by an inherited mutation in the tumor suppressor gene p53 and increases patients' risk for many different cancers, including breast cancer. Muir-Torre syndrome is caused by an inherited mutation of the DNA mismatch repair genes, in particular MSH2 and MLH1, which leads to an increased risk of colon and breast cancer.

In breast-ovary cancer syndrome, an inherited mutation in one of the two copies of either the gene BRCA-1 or the gene BRCA-2 is associated with a 50- to 85-percent lifetime risk of breast cancer. Recent laboratory tests suggest that BRCA-1 acts as a tumor suppressor and helps in the process of repairing damaged DNA in cells.

The general pattern in inherited female breast cancer syndromes is that the first of several mutations that can lead to cancer is present at birth, and it appears to enhance the tendency of breast cells to develop additional mutations.

We know that, for all women, the risk of breast cancer increases with age from about 1 in 20,000 women by age 25 to 1 in 9 by age 85. Presumably, this has to with the increasing chance of genetic injury in breast tissue cells as you grow older. The incidence in cancer is also much higher in Western countries like the United States, than in Asian countries, like Japan. Women who move from low-risk countries to high-risk countries have an increased risk of getting breast cancer, which suggests that environmental factors may play a significant role. A series of other factors related to uninterrupted ovulation, like beginning your menstrual period early, entering menopause late in life, having no children, or having your first full-term pregnancy after age 30, all increase the risk of breast cancer.

What the Future Holds for Breast Cancer Treatment

Basic science and clinical research have resulted in significant advances in both the understanding of the biology of breast cancer and treatment. Recent developments hold the promise of great strides in prevention and care in any stage of this disease. New therapies currently undergoing testing include anti-angiogenesis agents, which block the formation of new blood vessels that are essential for tumor growth, signal transduction inhibitors, which target aberrant growth or survival signals inside the cancer cell, and gene therapy approaches, which seem to be most useful currently in creating a tumor vaccine from some of the patient's own cancer cells.

CHAPTER ELEVEN

Radiotherapy: What to Know, What to Ask

By Bernard S. Lewinsky, M.D., F.A.C.R.

Radiation therapy has been used for breast cancer for well over a hundred years, since the discovery of the X ray by Konrad Roentgen in 1895. A Chicago chemist Emil Grubé was working on this same discovery, but the ship carrying his treatise was delayed by a winter storm and did not reach the scientific congress in Germany in time to be presented. Thus, the only scientist submitting a scientific paper on this discovery was Roentgen who received all the recognition. Emile Grubé, however, treated the first patient with advanced breast cancer in January 1896, just a few weeks after the X ray was "discovered." He described the beneficial effects of the treatment on this patient, although they were only temporary.

Dramatic changes in radiation therapy have since taken place, and women today must not only be given the option for breast conservation in most cases, but must also be aware of the treatment options that are available for multiple conditions. This chapter addresses the important radiotherapeutic issues with which every patient should be acquainted in the management of her particular condition. Understanding the terms and rationale for treatment will alleviate fear. Understanding your options will empower you and make the treatment more tolerable.

Radiation Oncology and Radiation Oncologists

Radiation oncology is the field of medicine that treats malignancies with radiation alone or sometimes in addition to drugs or surgery. A radiation oncologist is a physician who is trained to treat cancers with radiation. He or she should be board-certified in the field as a specialist. The reason patients should be seen by a radiation oncologist is that no single specialist is versed in all of the details of the various modalities; the opinion to treat or not to treat should be made by a specialist in that field. Each field in oncology is extremely complex, and it is very difficult to practice in more than one area proficiently. In some institutions, such as breast programs or academic institutions, all specialists are in one location and can participate in the decision-making together. If, however, you live in a community where this form of consultative service is not available, you should consult a radiation oncologist to get his or her expert opinion about use of radiation in your particular situation. Patients are best served when they can discuss all aspects of their care at the outset of their illness, and they are better able to prepare mentally for the task of treatments when they have knowledge of what lies ahead.

The most common question patients ask in an initial consultation is, "If my surgeon says that 'he got it all' and the pathology states that all of the margins are clear, why do I need radiation therapy?" The answer is neither the surgeon nor the pathologist can see all of the cancer. Imagine that the cancer is like an octopus with an obvious head and very long fingers. The visible tumor is the head of the octopus, and the obvious arms of the octopus are the parts of the tumor that are seen as strands. The ends of the fingers stretch out long distances, and at the ends, the single cells intermingle within normal tissues. These miniscule cells are obviously not visible to the surgeon or pathologist. Thus, isolated cancer cells invisible to all methods of detection may linger in the breast or chest wall tissues after surgery.

Many studies have been done to test the hypothesis that the surgeon has indeed removed all of the cancer. Patients were randomized to receive radiation or no radiation. They were then followed closely. In those patients who did not receive radiation, the recurrence rate ranged from 38 to 50 percent. Ninety percent of the recurrences were in the same location where the primary tumor was originally found. It obviously does not matter how old a patient is; this principle is the same. Understanding this simplified explanation, which generally applies to every patient, makes the role of radiation more obvious.

Radiation

Radiation is a form of energy. We are accustomed to experiencing various forms of energy—light, color, sound, ultraviolet, radio waves, sonar, infrared, and radiation to name a few types. The frequency and wavelength define the different characteristics of each of these forms of energy. The energy of the wave depends on the number of wave peaks per a given distance. If you imagine a rope tied to a tree and that you are holding the other end of the rope, you see that you need to put energy into the rope to make it move up and down. The more waves you want in that piece of rope, the more energy that you must exert. Thus, some of the waves will be of more or less energy than others.

Radiation used in medicine comes from two major sources: if it is created in a machine or an X-ray tube, it is called an X ray; if the energy comes from a natural material, such as cobalt or uranium, the energy is called a gamma ray (or alpha or beta). The quality of the radiation is defined by its energy (number of waves per length). If a gamma ray has the same energy as the X ray, the two types of radiation are identical.

Today, most of the medical equipment used in cancer therapy is produced by linear accelerators of varying energies. The most commonly used energies for the treatment of breast cancer are between 1.2 to 6 mV (million electron volts). For very large breasts, a 10-mV beam is sometimes used.

How Is Radiation Given and How Does It Work?

Radiation treatment practices have been established for many years. Radiation is given on a daily basis, five days per week, until a certain dose has been delivered to the tissues. The daily doses and the total doses have become fairly standard throughout the world, and most facilities have accepted the standards and treat cancer in the same manner. There is no evidence that the radiation that is used to treat cancer causes new cancers.

The patient will usually come to the radiation department on a daily basis, lie down on a treatment couch, and receive treatment to the area of the breast or chest wall for a total of a few minutes.

How exactly does the radiation kill the cancer cell? Radiation is a beam of energy, and energy causes a change in the cancer cell that will prevent it from duplicating. A cancer cell that does not replicate itself dies. In order to be affected, the cancer cell must be in a "vulnerable" state—that is, the DNA of the cell must be formed in order to be subject to damage from radiation. This occurs most often when the cell is in the synthesis or mitosis stage. The energy (in this case radiation) beam can damage the DNA by directly hitting it (this is called a *direct hit*) or it can damage the DNA indirectly by creating an environment that disturbs the DNA. The latter scenario is more common. The energy beam causes water in the body to split into free radicals, which then will attack the DNA and cause it to split. This happens to both normal and cancer cells alike but, fortunately, normal cells can repair the damage while cancer cells are not able to repair; thus they die.

The basic mechanism described above explains several points that are important to understand. The constant repair of the normal cells that takes place within five to six hours after each treatment explains why patients may get tired from the treatments even though there is no sensation whatsoever while the treatment is being delivered. It takes a lot of energy to repair normal cells. Secondly, the formation of free radicals to damage the DNA of the cancer cells might be hindered if the patient is taking antioxidants while the radiation is being delivered. Antioxidants trap free radicals. There are no clear-cut studies to prove this absolutely, but there is evidence that taking antioxidants, high-dose vitamin C, selenium, or other such compounds may be counterproductive to radiation therapy. Because these are not essential compounds, it is recommended that they not be taken during the course of radiation.

Lumpectomy/Radiation versus Mastectomy

There is a sentiment among many patients, and sometimes physicians, that removing the breast (mastectomy) will provide a better chance for a cure. However, there is data available now from almost every corner of the world that refutes this belief. There is *no survival* advantage to a mastectomy. In other words, how you treat the breast does not affect survival because if the tumor has spread elsewhere in the body, the local treatment—that is, removal of the tumor by surgery or radiation—is not the most important parameter. However, when the tumor has not spread, then the local treatment becomes most important. The equal alternative treatment to mastectomy is removal of the tumor (lumpectomy) plus irradiation of the breast. Thus, the price for keeping the breast is a course of radiation therapy. Careful surveillance of the irradiated breast is necessary as there is a small chance that the tumor could escape the effects of the radiation and recur locally. The incidence of local recurrence is approximately 7 to 15 percent at five years with lumpectomy and radiation. Obtaining wide margins of clearance is critical to maintaining low rates of local recurrence after lumpectomy or mastectomy. When mastectomy is performed, there is still a two- to nine-percent chance or so for a recurrence of the tumor in the chest wall area. There is no treatment that will give a perfect result. For these reasons, the cure of cancer is dependent on its spread. The primary function of the oncologist, whether medical, radiation, or surgical, is to analyze every aspect of risk of spread to provide appropriate treatment.

New techniques for delivering the radiation to the area where the tumor once was are currently being studied. These techniques include placing radioactive materials in the cavity or in the tissues surrounding the removed tumor. The early results from a handful of studies are promising, and in the next few years, the treatment methods after lumpectomy may change quite dramatically.

Stage, Size, and Histology of the Tumor

The size of the tumor, the number of lymph nodes involved, and the presence of tumor elsewhere in the body are factors used to stage the tumor. The purpose of staging a tumor is to be able to predict outcome and the risk of a recurrence. The histology of the tumor represents the type of tumor and the possible behavior of that tumor. All of these factors are important in deciding whether or not to irradiate, where to irradiate, and what dose to use. Many combinations of the above three factors can lead to different doses and areas of treatment.

There are certain (histology) types of tumor that may not require a course of radiation. These are tumors of special histology with features that are an exception and not the norm. Your radiation oncologist will discuss these with you, but be aware that the vast majority of patients who do not undergo mastectomy will require radiation treatments, except for those rare patients with tumors with special features or those with other unusual circumstances, which will be discussed later in this chapter.

Invasive versus Noninvasive Tumors

Invasive or *noninvasive* refers to whether a tumor has grown into surrounding tissues or whether it is confined to the structure from which it arose. For example, if the tumor is confined to the duct and has not grown into the surrounding tissues, it is called *in situ tumor*. Because it comes from a duct, it is called *ductal carcinoma in situ* (DCIS). If the tumor has begun to invade other tissue, then it is called *invasive ductal carcinoma*.

For the most part, invasive cancer treated by lumpectomy requires radiation whereas some forms of DCIS may not require radiation in addition to lumpectomy. The latter point is a very controversial issue, and not all physicians are in agreement. You will have to discuss this issue with your radiation oncologist. Several studies suggest that not every form of DCIS requires radiation treatment after lumpectomy. National trials are under way to test this hypothesis. Certainly, there appear to be differences among varieties of DCIS. Thus, there may well be groups of tissue types and tumor sizes that can be removed with adequate margins and so do not require further treatment. Hopefully, the studies will answer these questions.

Radiation for Early-Stage Disease

The notion that early, small tumors of the invasive variety do not need to be treated with radiation also exists. The idea that a small tumor can be removed more completely than a larger tumor, negating the need for radiation, has been tested by randomized studies. Once again, studies addressing the issue of local control showed that surgery alone was insufficient for the vast majority of tumors. Radiation is needed to sterilize the area.

Radiation for Late-Stage Disease

When the cancer in the breast is very large or there are many positive lymph nodes, the risk for tumor spread is so high that the local treatment must take a secondary role at the start of treatment. Eventually the local tumor will have to be treated by either surgery alone or with the combination of surgery and radiation. Chemotherapy may be instituted first to treat the potential tumor that may have spread and will most likely have an effect on the primary tumor. Most likely, the tumor will reduce in size while the chemotherapy is administered. If the tumor responds, a surgical procedure will ultimately remove the tumor area, and radiation will then be given to prevent the cancer from growing further in the breast. The more advanced the tumor, the higher the dose of radiation needed to control the tumor. Neoadjuvant therapy (treatment before surgery with chemotherapy or radiation therapy) is a controversial issue that may or may not be relevant to you.

Even when mastectomy is performed, radiation to treat the chest wall is required when the tumor is greater than four centimeters or when there are multiple positive lymph nodes. Several studies have shown the benefit of post-mastectomy radiation in terms of survival advantage. When the tumor or stage of cancer is advanced, radiation is given to sterilize the local area.

Integrating Radiation with Chemotherapy

It has been shown that chemotherapy should be given within two months of surgery to be most effective. Adding radiation at the same time increases the side effects of both treatments and depletes the bone marrow of white cells, potentially causing a delay in chemotherapy because of the patient's low white blood cell count or because of the increased skin reactions due to the interaction of chemotherapy with radiation. Chemotherapy is usually given before radiation because the greatest risk to the patient if cancer cells have spread elsewhere is delay of treatment to those areas, which is the main purpose of chemotherapy. If, however, chemotherapy is given for a longer period than four to six months, the risk of *local* recurrence begins to increase. Neither of these situations is ideal.

The oncology team usually discusses their approach to these issues and coordinates the delivery of the two modalities. You should be aware of the facts and be prepared to question your physician about the timing of the two treatments. On very few occasions, both chemotherapy and radiation therapy are given together. Some chemotherapy drugs affect the response to radiation (for example, they make the skin burn more readily) and thus only certain drugs can be given in combination with radiation.

Treatment Area and Administration of Radiation

If a mastectomy is performed, the entire breast is removed; when the breast is not removed, the entire breast must be treated. Breasts have varying sizes, shapes, contours, and amounts of fatty tissue, but they all lie uniformly in front of the ribs on the chest wall. The patient lies on a treatment table with her arm placed in a position that exposes the entire chest area. The treatment machine is turned and the area of radiation is determined so as to encompass the breast and chest wall. This procedure is known as the *simulation*—that is, the treatment is planned but not executed. Frequently a computerized scan (CT, or CAT scan) is utilized to clearly delineate the breast in relation to the chest wall and

WHAT ARE THE RADIATION DOSIMETRIST'S QUALIFICATIONS?

A radiation dosimetrist is trained to generate a plan that will treat the tumor as uniformly as possible with the aid of sophisticated planning programs. The radiation oncologist will provide the dosimetrist with the anatomical structures to be treated (or those to be spared). The dosimetrist will then develop an appropriate plan

the targeted lymph nodes. The chest wall is a curved structure with the lungs lying directly beneath the ribs. On the left side, there may be a portion of the heart, but since gravity pulls the heart downwards in the supine position, the majority of the heart should *not* be in the treatment area. The central portion of the chest is the mediastinum and just adjacent to the sternum are another set of lymph nodes, internal mammary lymph nodes, that occasion-

ally need to be treated. These structures vary in the exact location and size from patient to patient, thus requiring an individual plan for each treated area. You can, and perhaps should, ask to be shown the final plans so that you are involved in the process of your treatment. Let me emphasize that the radiation oncologist should minimize the amount of normal tissues included in the treatment field but must also be cognizant of the pattern of spread and the statistical risk for each individual patient. For example, a patient with very large breasts may pose a great challenge for the physician and, on very few occasions, if there is no alternative way to minimize the normal tissue included (mainly the heart), the patient may not be a candidate for the conventional type of radiation. If this is your situation, you may have to be treated facedown with your breast suspended through an opening to allow the treatment machine to deliver the radiation to the breast in that position. If it's not possible to protect the heart, lungs, and other structures adequately, you may not be a candidate for whole breast radiation. It's possible that localized treatments will become more standard for women in these situations.

The areas of treatment are known as *fields*. There usually are two fields that treat the breast: the medial and lateral fields. One-half of the daily dose is given from each field. This arrangement delivers a uniform distribution of the radiation inside the breast. The radiation dosimetrist is a person specifically trained to prepare a plan on a computer that delineates the radiation patterns within the area of the body that is being treated. The radiation oncologist then selects the most appropriate plan for the patient.

New methods to try to isolate the radiation to the actual breast tissue are being developed with the hope of sparing the normal tissues that do not need to be irradiated. These methods may or may not turn out to be useful. For example, the treatments will become so complex and take so much time to deliver that the value and outcome of such precise technology may not be feasible from the logistics of therapy.

WHO WILL DELIVER YOUR RADIATION THERAPY?

The radiation therapist is the person who will deliver your prescribed treatments. The radiation therapist, who has been trained by an approved institution, is the right-hand person of the radiation oncologist. He or she will play a very important role in your care, recording the doses of radiation and monitoring the doses on a daily basis. The radiation therapist becomes your advocate during the period of treatment. Your radiation oncologist's staff should be compassionate, kind, accurate, and professional.

Once the area, field size, and treatment plan are set, the treatment can be given. The patient lies in the same position, the fields are set up daily, and the dose of radiation is delivered. The actual treatment time varies according to the equipment manufacturer, the dose, the physics of the plan, and so forth. It usually lasts two to three minutes per area. Setup time takes the longest; the delivery is rather short. There is no sensation whatsoever while the radiation is delivered. The patient then comes off the treatment table and can go on with the rest of her/his day.

Indications against Radiation Treatment

There are only a few contraindications preventing a patient from becoming a candidate for breast-saving surgery and radiation therapy:

• Collagen vascular disease, such as scleroderma. The tissues do not tolerate radiation because of the basic nature of the disease.

• Multiple suspicious calcifications throughout the breast, suggesting multiple or extensive tumors.

- More than one tumor in the breast, unless they are close to each other and can be removed with an extended lumpectomy or quadrantectomy.

- Previous radiation for Hodgkin's disease.

- Social and medical factors that disallow adequate delivery or follow-up.

Treatment of the Lymph Nodes in the Axilla

The lymph nodes are sometimes involved with the cancerous process. The radiation fields that are applied to the breast usually treat the lower levels of lymph nodes because, anatomically, the lower lymph nodes are in close proximity to the breast. However, there are times when the statistical probability that additional nodes may be involved with cancer is so high that treatment of the higher levels of nodes must be given. A field separate from the breast tangents that encompasses the upper lymph nodes is given. Adding other areas increases the side effects of therapy very slightly, but the recurrence of tumor in that area carries a much more severe consequence. Thus, this field is sometimes treated to ensure control of that region.

The indications for treating the additional axillary field are rather well-defined in the literature. These include:

- Multiple lymph nodes (more than three or four) were positive in the nodes that were sampled.

- The lymph nodes that were positive had very extensive growth outside the boundaries of the node. This is known as *extra capsular extension.*

- There is extensive lymph channel involvement seen under the microscope.

- There are unusual factors that increase the risk for involvement in that area.

The most serious side effect of treating the axilla (underarm) is swelling (edema) of the arm following treatment. The swelling may be in part related to the surgery, but the combination of the two (surgery and radiation) may be the cause of the edema. Fortunately, the incidence of edema is quite low with the more limited amount of axillary surgery being performed today. The extent of edema may vary from mild tightness of the wrist and fingers to swelling that requires a compression sleeve to reduce the edema. Again, the risk of cancer recurrence must be weighed against the risk of arm or hand swelling. The former has much more serious consequences.

Under very special circumstances, the internal mammary lymph nodes, which are adjacent to the sternum, must also be treated. They are irradiated with special techniques designed to avoid treating the heart and underlying structure of the mediastinum.

What Is a Boost and When Do You Use It?

A boost is an additional dose given through a reduced field size that encompasses the area where the tumor was first taken out. Data have shown that most recurrences take place in the same location where the tumor was initially discovered. The largest concentrations of residual cancer cells are located near the tumor site and thus a higher dose of radiation is needed to sterilize that region. A recent European study compared "boosts" to "no boosts." After adequate follow-up in the study, the patients who were "boosted" had a significantly lower rate of recurrence. Consequently, most patients will receive a boost. The boost adds five to eight additional treatments to the smaller area after the entire breast has been treated. Usually the boost area becomes slightly more irritated with slightly more skin reaction, such as itching, peeling, redness, or skin burning. As in other areas, these reactions subside within a few weeks after treatment.

External beams (either X rays or electrons) are used for the boost. However, there are occasions when a cancer was very close to the margin or where additional surgery was not feasible due to the anatomical location. Then, an internal boost can be given. This is known as an *interstitial* (inside the tissue) *implant*. Plastic catheters are placed inside the breast in the appropriate area under local anesthesia or light anesthesia. The tubes remain in the breast and are a vehicle for placing radioactive materials inside the breast temporarily. The material is left in place until a specified dose is delivered. Due to the physics of radiation, the intensity inside the breast is higher and thus a more effective dose is given that can sterilize the area. This procedure, however, requires a minor surgical procedure. It is usually done on an inpatient basis, but depending on the method of delivering the radiation, you may also be treated as an outpatient.

> During radiation, I followed the doctor's advice using a preparation that contained no alcohol. I used aloe vera three times a day, and I didn't burn badly because I followed their instructions. Radiation therapy did make me feel tired, especially getting to the treatments, because I had to drive great lengths. • Linda R.

> I was very burned, but at night, I would get gel ice packs and wrap them around my side, making sure that the ice pack didn't touch my skin, and that helped. • Cynthia

> My situation was very unusual, I had radiation a second time, and that was real tough. But for most people it doesn't hurt. Take good care of your skin with aloe. • Joelle

Side Effects of Radiation

The side effects of radiation treatments can take place during the treatments. These are called *acute reactions*. They may also occur at a later time when they are referred to as *delayed* or *chronic reactions*. Remember, this is a seven-week treatment. Acute reactions that almost always take place are fatigue, skin reactions, which may be minor or intense, itching of the skin, and minor breakout of skin rash. Occasionally patients also have some swelling during the treatments. There is usually no hair loss or nausea and vomiting related to treatment of the breast area. Most of the side effects can be managed by the use of topical medications that your doctor should prescribe or tell you about.

Some topical preparations contain alcohol and/or perfumes and may actually increase the intensity of the reaction. The best preparations are moisturizing creams that contain no alcohol or perfume, such as Eucerin or Aquafor. Once the itching starts, some topical one percent hydrocortisone will be useful. Aloe vera, either in plant form or extract, is very soothing to the skin and can be used during the entire course of treatment. Bathing with tepid water and mild soap is helpful and necessary.

If your breasts are large or have too many folds as they attach to the chest wall, the radiation beam will bounce in the folds, creating a more intense reaction that may actually break down the skin temporarily. Hot climate usually increases the reactions. It may be helpful to refrain from wearing a bra during that period of time. Wearing absorbent clothes such as cotton will be helpful, because synthetic materials are not as absorbent, and moisture will increase the reaction. If the reaction becomes very uncomfortable, ice packs and topical steroids may also help. Your physician or radiation nurse can advise you on how to best manage your reactions. By far, the greatest complaint I get from patients regarding the treatments is the traffic to and from the treatment!

The long-term or chronic side effects may take one to two years to develop and may be more long lasting. The most common changes are:

- Edema (swelling) of the breast

- Edema of the arms

- Skin pigmentation

- Retraction of the breast (shrinkage of the ligaments that suspend the breast)

- The texture and softness of the skin

- The development of small red vessels called *telangiectasia*

Because radiation therapy for the intact breast is basically given to save the breast, one would like to be able to get a result in which there is absolutely no difference between the two breasts. Unfortunately, this is not realistic, although it can sometimes happen. The cosmetic results of therapy are usually excellent, but not perfect. Your healing processes are mostly responsible for the eventual outcome. There may be a small cosmetic price to pay by keeping the breast, but it is undoubtedly far better than the best reconstructed breast. The breast is also sensate (the breast and nipples have sensation and can play a role in sexual arousal), whereas the reconstructed breast will not have sensation. However, if reconstruction is necessary, or you choose mastectomy and reconstruction, an experienced plastic and reconstructive surgeon can be consulted.

Incidentally, it's sometimes necessary to irradiate a reconstructed breast for oncological reasons. We would do this to sterilize the chest wall area in order to try to prevent recurrence on the chest wall covered with the new breast. Depending on the technique used, a reconstructed breast will tolerate the radiation quite well.

Edema of the breast occurs as a result of the disruption of the lymph channels in the tissues by either surgery or radiation. By and large, the acute edema disappears within a few months, but sometimes it takes one to two years to dissipate completely. My advice is always to wait rather than to do corrective procedures too soon—for example, breast reductions or tissue flap advancement—as the problems usually resolve with time.

Skin pigmentation is the result of the effect of radiation on the skin. The melanin-producing cells are stimulated to produce pigment, and the pigmentation may remain permanently in some people. The color differences vary from very subtle to obvious.

Breast retraction is mainly due to the shrinkage of ligaments that suspend the breast to their original level. Pregnancy and breast-feeding stretch the ligaments causing breasts to sag; radiation brings the ligaments back to the original state. Most women love their irradiated breasts. But we do not treat the other to make them match, so there will be a difference between the two breasts.

The small vessels that may develop on the skin of the irradiated breast are of no significant consequence to most patients. Occasionally they are associated with itching of the skin. Normally they are just nuisances. They do, however, relate to the degree of injury to the normal skin from the radiation and are a sign that the skin has been injured and that further injury, such as surgery, could be accompanied by delayed healing and ulceration. In general, it's advisable to approach surgery on the irradiated breast with extreme caution, as we don't know how an individual will heal under those circumstances.

Occasionally scar tissue will develop in the high-dose radiation area. With time, this scar tissue may be firm and tender and can be confused with recurrence of cancer. It is either fat tissue breakdown (yes, the majority of the breast is fatty tissue), or it may be a scar. The value of mammograms and biopsies is that they can usually differentiate these conditions. Follow-up care is needed to understand the process of each individual patient in order not to miss early detection of tumor recurrence. Biopsy in the radiated breast is best done by core needle biopsy, fine needle aspiration, or, if necessary, a small surgery biopsy meticulously performed.

There are a number of chronic side effects that occur in a very small percentage of people. Listing all of these would require a lengthy chapter and may not be exhaustive because every patient may respond to treatment in a slightly different way. The important side reactions must be understood and the others left to discussion if necessary. After all, most physicians recommend therapy because it is needed for the treatment of the malignancy. Recurrence of cancer is a much more risky proposition. The best treatment is always the first treatment and if you become totally entrenched in the details of side effects without taking into account the incidence, you will have a very difficult time accepting recommendations for treatments.

Who Should Follow You after You Have Completed Your Treatments? Why the Radiation Oncologist Also?

Certainly, from the point of view of the body as a whole, the medical oncologist should be involved in the aftercare program, especially if he or she has given chemotherapy. The radiation oncologist also contributes to the follow-up program because he or she examines you with the knowledge of the given treatment and the possible changes that radiation can cause in the breast. This is an area of oncology that is very important, yet some patients have a hard time understanding why the medical and radiation oncologist who treated them should follow them.

(Any suspicion of local recurrence should immediately involve the appropriate surgeon.)

An example may illustrate this point. A woman was treated with a course of radiation therapy. She had a residual firmness after the biopsy, which remained after her treatments. I observed the presence of these findings and recorded them in my notes. She changed insurance, as happens frequently today, to an HMO that did not allow follow-up by specialists. (Not all HMOs have the same guidelines.) New doctors, who had not previously examined her, saw her. They brought up the issue of possible cancer recurrence. She was advised to have that area removed and, being in a panicked state, agreed. The new physicians removed the same area of firmness that I had noted in my previous records. No cancer was found since it was residual scar tissue from her first surgery. The surgery was not necessary. Had I been told of the surgeon's suspicions I could have advised him against surgery that damaged her cosmetic result and her psyche. My advice is that the medical and radiation oncologists should follow the patient, if at all possible, with reasonable intervals. Each specialist inherently sees through the eyes of his or her specialty, and the result is a benefit to the patient.

What Can Be Done If the Cancer Recurs in the Breast or Chest Wall after Radiation Therapy?

Generally when there is a local recurrence after primary radiation therapy following lumpectomy, mastectomy is the only recommendation given. The results obtained with these primary treatments obviously vary with tumor size and nodal status, but, in general, local control is very high as long as the surgeon obtains good margins of clearance during the lumpectomy. There are no new technologies at present to deal with recurrences with radiation because the doses delivered initially are usually high. But not all situations are identical; thus all options should be reevaluated.

Recurrence of tumor after postmastectomy chest wall irradiation can sometimes be dealt with by local treatment with microwave hyperthermia and low doses of radiation and surgical excision when possible. Unfortunately, hyperthermia has not become standard in the majority of institutions and may not be an option for everyone. Local small-field reirradiation is sometimes possible. A rapid local recurrence (within two years) of the chest wall after radiation, however, carries a guarded prognosis since it usually heralds the appearance of cancer elsewhere. Each case must be dealt with individually, and no general statements can be made that apply to everyone. Usually chemotherapy is used alone or in combination with local radiation or surgery.

If the Cancer Has Spread

When cancer has spread, or metastasized, radiation can be used to decrease cancerous areas in other parts of the body. Chemotherapy is usually the main treatment, but when an area is particularly painful, such as the bone, local, short courses of radiation can eliminate the pain and allow for a decreased use of strong pain medication. Most organs can be treated for palliation (pain control) except the liver, which does not tolerate radiation well. The doses are very small and insufficient to have an effect on the cancer itself.

Radiation can be given to control cancer that has spread to the brain. Hair loss is the unfortunate effect of this treatment. Usual doses delivered to the brain do not affect mental function in the short term. Usually patients with brain tumors are quite symptomatic, and the change for the better in mental function is usually quite welcome. Over a long period of time—that is, five years or more—there may be residual slowing of the thought processes such as addition and subtraction done mentally.

In Summary

If you are planning radiation therapy, remember that radiation therapy has been in use for over a hundred years and that it is well-tolerated with relatively few side effects. Your radiation oncologist is an important member of your treatment team and should be consulted early in the post-diagnosis period. The radiation oncologist also plays an important role in your after-treatment care. When planning radiotherapy, you must be proactive. Be absolutely sure that you understand all aspects of your treatment. Ask questions until you do!

CHAPTER TWELVE

Behind the Microscope: The Critical Role of the Pathologist

By William J. Colburn, M.D.

A diagnosis of cancer brings with it many difficult emotions. In addition, there is the difficulty of being labeled as having "cancer" with its attendant risk to life and limb as well as the added burden of having to sift through the rather bewildering and enormously complex issues concerning your treatment choices. The pathologist can only imagine what you may be going through knowing that, because of his or her rendered tissue diagnosis, your life has been inexorably altered. Yet many of the treatment choices you will have to make are based upon the pathologist's evaluation of your biopsy, and it is my contention that the pathologist is well-suited to help you understand your disease and its prognostic implications.

What a Pathologist Does

A pathologist studies tissues, and the breast pathologist is a physician trained to evaluate an array of breast pathology specimens, including fine needle aspiration biopsies, surgical breast biopsies of all types, lymph nodes, and ultimately mastectomies. (For the purposes of this chapter, we'll focus on the surgical removal of a mass or tissue density.)

The pathologist's evaluation of your cancer plays a pivotal role in diagnosis and treatment decisions. The characteristics of your tumor (and removed lymph nodes) help us to determine the stage of your disease and what treatment choices are likely to be most effective. Traditionally your oncologist or surgeon has assumed the role of mentor to help you understand your disease and prognosis, but the pathologist is the physician most familiar with the scope and extent of your illness and should readily accept the challenge of serving not only as diagnostician but also as a guide and mentor.

Evaluating Your Specimen: From the Operating Room to the Laboratory

Before consulting with you, your pathologist should be aware of the clinical and mammographic findings that led to your formal biopsy. This must be done through the efforts of a coordinated biopsy team, usually comprised of the pathologist, surgeon, and radiologist. Many patients will have had a fine needle aspiration or core needle biopsy that has shown cancer or atypia (abnormal cell growth). In these cases, particularly, it is mandatory that the pathologist be in the operating room when your cancer is removed to know its exact location in the breast and to maintain its three-dimensional orientation to later aid in the determination that the margins are free of tumor.

If localization wires were placed into your breast preoperatively, the pathologist should conduct the specimen to the radiology department for specimen X ray. Specimen radiology should be performed under the direction of a radiologist and in the presence of the pathologist, who will continue to be in charge of maintaining its proper orientation as it is taken from one department to the other. The biopsy specimen is X-rayed to determine whether the proper area has been removed and that the margins appear to be adequate. The specimen should never be passed between multiple radiologists and pathologists, as this only increases the chance of processing a tissue specimen for microscopic evaluation after anatomic orientation has been irretrievably lost.

The tissue biopsy specimen is next taken to the pathology laboratory, where its outer margins are dyed with different colored inks so

| WHY YOU NEED AN EXPERT PATHOLOGIST

The pathologist's ability to perform immediate frozen section is a very subjective and difficult task, requiring sophisticated training, talent, and significant expertise. An expert breast pathologist can accurately assess your margins of clearance and other biological characteristics of your cancer.

The pathologist's ability to determine the margins of clearance (the amount of normal breast tissue between the edge of the cancer and the edge of the lumpectomy) is extremely important to the outcome of your surgery. Knowing whether you have clear margins, and by how many millimeters is a crucial aspect of cancer care. If you don't get a clean margin, you will need additional surgery. Further, widely clear margins can reduce the possibility of a recurrence of cancer in the treated area.

Seek the services of a pathologist who is interested in and committed to breast pathology. Breast cancer care is a team effort, requiring the coordinated consultation of a top-level breast surgeon and pathologist, among many other specialists. An expert breast surgeon will most likely work in collaboration with a very experienced pathologist. You can learn more about choosing a quality pathologist in Chapter 19, "How to Get the Best Breast Cancer Care and Treatment."

that, upon final microscopic evaluation, six tissue planes of excision, at a minimum, can be evaluated for tumoral clearance. The six planes of excision refer to anatomically oriented margins of resection (the edges of the removed tissue)—that is, anterior (subcutaneous or skin), deep (toward the chest muscle), lateral (toward the arm), medial (toward the center/midline of the body), superior (toward the head), and inferior (toward the feet).

If a suspicious mass or tumor is noted, a frozen section will be performed. This entails taking a piece of the mass and placing it in a machine called a *Cryostat.* The tissue is frozen. Then, ultrathin sections (about the thickness of a human hair) are cut and placed on a slide. The slide is removed from the machine and stained with a supravital dye so that the pathologist can look at the cellular details of the mass under the microscope. The microscopic findings are discussed with the surgeon while you are asleep in the operating room. If a cancer is diagnosed, the pathologist will further describe the preliminary microscopic finding of the malignancy with the surgeon and advise the surgeon whether the tumor has been adequately removed—that is to say, whether the entire tumor is located within the specimen, its relationship to all of the margins of resection (the removed area), and how far the tumor is from each respective margin (in millimeters). The establishment of a tumor-free margin of approximately five to ten millimeters in all directions is considered to be an adequate lumpectomy. In most instances, getting adequate margins will result in a substantial decrease in the possibility of a recurrence at the area from which the tumor was removed. No tissue should be discarded and any remaining biopsy should be preserved in 10 percent formalin fixative or paraffin embedded, should further microscopic tissue evaluation or special studies be required for any reason.

Now the pathologist can begin to perform the most important phase of total biopsy procedure, which encompasses tissue processing for microscopic evaluation and final histological (microanatomic) examination. Final pathology results are typically available in one to three days postoperatively.

The Pathology Report

A standardized surgical pathology report paints a word picture of the removed tissue—for example, a tumor removed from the breast and axillary lymph node contents. It is usually divided into components, which includes the gross tissue description. The gross tissue description refers to the tumor as it is seen with the naked eye. At the very minimum, the gross tissue description should contain information about the type of specimen and its location within the breast; the measurements of its three dimensions before formalin fixation and sectioning; the weight of the specimen, if relevant; a written description of the tissue, including the size, color, consistency, and contour of the lesion (tumor) and the relationship of the tumor to its inked margins; radiographic findings of the X ray of the tissue specimen and its correlation to mammographic views of the breast; and a summary tissue legend, which should state which tissue sections are contained in which individually labeled tissue cassettes (small containers for tissue slices). Small biopsy specimens should be submitted in their entirety in up to five tissue

| EVALUATING THE SENTINEL LYMPH NODE

The chapter "Removing Lymph Nodes" outlays the rationale behind surgical treatment of the lymph nodes in the armpit (axilla) and about newer techniques that allow for the detection of the sentinel node. Axillary staging is used to direct your course of treatment after surgery, as clinical trials have demonstrated prolonged survival for node-positive women who are treated with adjuvant chemotherapy and hormone therapy. The sentinel node is the first node that drains a specific area of the body—in this case, the breast. It is the node within the axilla most likely to harbor metastatic breast cancer cells.

If you have elected to receive sentinel node and/or additional lymph node dissection, the pathologist will evaluate the sentinel node at the time of surgery. This process consists of performing a frozen section or touch preparation, which involves dabbing the cut surface of the lymph node onto a glass slide, staining it, and then reviewing the cells that have adhered to the slide with a microscope. In most cases, both frozen section and touch preparation are able to detect the presence of malignant tumor cells within the substances of the lymph node. The false negative rate for both procedures is approximately 10 to 15 percent. After frozen section, the frozen section tissue is placed in a fixative (usually 10 percent buffered formalin) and submitted for thorough microscopic evaluation to corroborate the initial frozen section/rapid smear results. An additional ultrasensitive test called *Immunohistochemistry (IHC)* is then employed to detect breast cancer micrometastasis (microscopic cancer spread) to the axillary lymph node. This is currently the most sensitive light microscope technique that the pathologist can employ. If the sentinel node is found negative by both light microscopic and ultrasensitive IHC technique for metastatic breast cancer, the probability of additional non-sentinel axillary lymph nodes being involved with carcinoma is less than one in a thousand per individual lymph node.

cassettes, and larger specimens should be sampled with at least two-thirds of the nonfatty tissue submitted for processing. There may be a separate description of the biopsy as seen under the microscope in unusual cases, but normally the information about the microscopic description is incorporated within the final microscopic evaluation and tissue diagnosis.

The final summary microscopic evaluation and histologic tissue analysis is the most important part of the pathology report and should outline the characteristics of your tumor, including whether or not it is invasive; its type, size, and biological features; ER/PR receptor status;

what the margins of clearance are; whether or not your cancer is linked to the overproduction of a growth factor called her2/neu (see Chapter 10, "Chemotherapy, Hormone Therapy, and the Stages of Breast Cancer"); and the status of your lymph nodes. (To learn how to read and interpret a pathology report, talk to your pathologist. Most pathologists are available to help patients understand their pathology reports.)

Armed with the final microscopic and summary anatomic pathology report, you can now consider seeking private consultation with a pathologist. This may be the original pathologist or an expert breast pathologist in the community. A pathologist should never solicit a consultation with a patient, and you shouldn't have to appear with check in hand. In 20 years of practice, I have performed more than five hundred personal pathology consultations, and I've never sought payment for these services, as they are a valued componenet of the total scope of anatomic pathology services rendered for the patient and/or for which her insurance has been previously billed.

If your biopsy was performed at an outside institution, you should bring all your pathology records and slides with you at the time of your appointment with the consulting pathologist. Your scheduled appointment should last a minimum of an hour in order to have time enough to conduct the review of your case at an unhurried pace. If needed, additional time can be scheduled. You should be encouraged to bring your significant other or important person with you. Bringing a trusted person with you can stimulate further questions and, most importantly, ensure that all parties "hear the same thing."

Usually you will have your consultation in the pathologist's office. It should be quiet and comfortable and free of extraneous noise and interruptions. The pathologist should have a multiheaded teaching microscope on hand so that everyone can look at the microscopic pathology in the same instance and in "real time." At the beginning of your session, the pathologist should briefly describe his or her role in the operating room and all other departments of the hospital to maintain the three-dimensional orientation of the specimen so vital to getting an authoritative histological/microscopic evaluation of your biopsy. You should learn how the specimen is described and sectioned and how, in general, tissue slides for microscopic evaluation are prepared. You should feel free to ask any questions you have, knowing that no question is "too simple" or "irrelevant." While I try to answer all questions to the best of my ability, I refrain from answering questions about the need for further adjuvant treatments as these are best posed to the treating physicians.

Next, I review the basic microanatomy of the female breast, usually using your own slide material for this purpose. It often helps to see that there is structurally normal tissue present and to look at the difference between normal and abnormal pathology. We can then proceed through a comprehensive review of the summary of the anatomic pathology histological analysis of the biopsy specimen. All of the terms on the report should be thoroughly discussed in clear language. I have found illustrations of the breast and its microanatomy to be very helpful in bringing the pathologist's "path-o-babble" into crystal clear focus. A simple sketch can also be useful. You may want to keep them for future reference. I also use a ruler in inches and millimeters to show the size of tumors and their distance from the inked margins of excision.

If the consulting pathologist is the pathologist who initially evaluated your biopsy, you may want to seek a second opinion. This should be encouraged. Your slides and printed material should be made readily available to you and should be released into your custody after signing a simple release form. You may want to ask for recommendations of expert breast pathologists, whose names should also be readily available to you. I typically end my sessions by telling patients that if they have any additional questions I would be most happy to answer them whenever they should arise. If further surgery has been scheduled, I make it a point to let the patient know that I will review any and all tissue materials and/or reports.

Your consultation should end on a positive note. You should have a clear understanding of your disease, hopefully with the information presented to you in an empathic and caring manner.

Educating Yourself

Understanding the nature of your tumor and pathologic findings can influence your decision for or against further adjuvant nonsurgical and/or surgical interventions. While you may speak to your medical oncologist or surgeon, the pathologist is in some ways the most familiar with your cancer at a cellular level and may be most equipped to help you understand its pathobiology, preparing you to ask the most cogent questions about therapeutic modalities offered by your treating physicians. You will have continued visits with your gynecologist, internist, medical oncologist, and, at times, your surgeon; a visit to your pathologist can be equally valuable and informative.

CHAPTER THIRTEEN

Anesthesia: What You Should Know before Surgery

By Howard Singer, M.D.

If you are planning breast surgery, you should be aware of the various options available for anesthesia. Three types of anesthesia may be used for breast surgery:

- Straight local anesthesia

- Local anesthesia with sedation

- General anesthesia

Minor Procedures: Straight Local Anesthesia

For minor breast procedures, such as stereotactic breast biopsies or superficial excisional breast biopsies, straight local anesthesia may be all that you need. A local anesthetic solution, such as lidocaine, will be injected directly into the area of concern to numb it, much as a dentist would numb your gums for dental work. After your local anesthetic, you may be able to feel certain sensations, such as pulling or tugging, but you should feel no pain in the area. If you are very nervous or anxious about your procedure, you may want to ask for intravenous sedation in addition to local anesthesia.

Local Anesthesia with Sedation

Local anesthesia with sedation is similar to straight local anesthesia except that you will be given sedative drugs through an intravenous infusion (IV) prior to the injection of the local anesthesia. Like straight local anesthesia, this method may be used for minor procedures, and depending on patients' and surgeons' preferences, for some breast biopsies. Usually an anesthesiologist will be present for the procedure and will remain during the operation. Before your surgery, the anesthesiologist will examine you and take a brief medical history from you. You may get a preoperative sedative through an IV prior to the beginning of your surgery that will relax you and make you slightly drowsy, and you may also receive an IV antibiotic. Then, just before the injection of the local anesthetic, you may be given a second medication, which will put you in a light sleep so that you won't feel the injection. You may be aware and relaxed during the procedure or in a "twilight sleep," depending on your preference and your surgeon's preference. The medication is short-acting and will wear off quickly after your surgery is finished. Your vital signs will be monitored with a blood pressure cuff on your arm, an EKG monitor, and a pulse oximeter on your fingers to measure your oxygen levels. You'll also probably be given a loose-fitting oxygen mask to breath from.

> If you are afraid of surgery because you're afraid you'll wake up or if you are afraid of nausea, you can ask your anesthesiologist, "What is your plan? What is your alternative plan in case that doesn't work for me?" You can be up front about it, because you need to know.
> • Joelle

> Make sure you investigate your anesthesiologist. Talk to him or her directly before surgery. I think it's almost as important to investigate your anesthesiologist as any other doctor; your anesthesiologist has your life in his or her hands. • Linda L.

I wanted to see the anesthesiologist because I weigh less than a hundred pounds. Medical professionals are extremely busy people. You have to remind them of your needs, especially if you are not average in height or weight. · Beverly

General Anesthesia for Extensive Breast Surgery

For more extensive breast surgery, such as deeper lumpectomies, mastectomies, and reconstruction, you will require general anesthesia. An anesthesiologist will meet with you preoperatively. You will get an IV started in your arm and be given a preoperative sedative. Before going to sleep, your monitors—(EKG, blood pressure cuff, and pulse oximeter)—will be put on, and you will breath oxygen for a few minutes. A medication that will put you to sleep will be given in your IV. This may cause some burning at the IV site, but it won't last long. For shorter procedures, you may continue to breathe from the oxygen mask, and you will be given a mixture of anesthetic gases with oxygen, which will keep you asleep. Alternatively, a laryngeal mask airway (L.M.A.) will be inserted into your mouth after you are asleep to deliver the anesthetic gas mixture. This allows the mask to be removed from your face and helps to keep the breathing passages open.

For longer or more extensive operations, you may be intubated, which involves inserting a breathing tube into your windpipe after you are asleep. This way your breathing can be better controlled with a ventilator, and you are protected from aspiration under these conditions. Aspiration is when the stomach contents regurgitate into the mouth and enter the lungs through the vocal cords. This happens because you lose your protective gag reflex under

CHOOSING AN ANESTHESIOLOGIST

You can choose your anesthesiologist, but you must make a specific request before your surgery. Otherwise, you will be given the anesthesiologist who is assigned to you. When choosing an anesthesiologist, consider:

- **The anesthesiologist's education and training.** The anesthesiologist must have trained in an approved residency in anesthesiology. He or she should be board-certified or board eligible.

- **Reputation.** Your surgeon will usually know good anesthesiologists.

anesthesia, which normally prevents vomitus from passing through your vocal cords. Because of the risk of aspiration, you will be asked to be *NPO,* which means nothing by mouth, for eight hours prior to your operation. Usually it's okay to take

Before surgery, one of your doctors should listen to your heart and lungs to make certain that you have no cardiac or respiratory abnormalities. A preoperative history and physical examination should be on your hospital chart prior to surgery.

any medications you might be on with a sip of water in the morning, but otherwise you will be asked not to eat or drink after midnight the night before your surgery, or for at least eight hours, if your surgery is in the afternoon. At the end of surgery, the anesthetic gases are turned off, and you will breath pure oxygen. As the gases are breathed out, you will awaken, but you will remain drowsy for a period of time, usually around 30 minutes. If you are having surgery to remove axillary lymph nodes, your anesthesiologist will avoid drugs that block neuromuscular function during this portion of the surgery because these lymph nodes are near two important nerves.

Side Effects of Anesthesia

Nausea and vomiting are the most common side effects of general anesthesia. If this occurs, or if you have a history of postoperative nausea, you can be given a medication to treat this, such as Zofran or Anzemet. Of course, there are more serious complications that can occur with general anesthesia, but these are quite rare.

After Surgery: In the Recovery Room

If you feel any pain after your operation, you may be given an IV pain medication. The narcotic drugs, such as Demerol or morphine, are the most effective in treating postoperative pain but may make you nauseous and drowsy. If the pain is less severe, you may be given a pain pill to take orally once you are awake enough. Morphine does have side effects, including severe nausea, vomiting, sedation, and respiratory depression. Alternatives to morphine include Vicodin and Darvocet and injectable Toradol, although the latter alternative may inhibit platelets and cause bleeding, among other side effects.

After surgery, you will usually be kept in the recovery room for an hour or until you are awake and alert enough to be discharged or admitted to the hospital, if you have had a mastectomy. In most cases, lumpectomy and axillary lymph node sampling are performed on an outpatient basis. Mastectomy is generally an inpatient procedure.

A recovery nurse will be with you to monitor your vital signs and take care of you. You should not drive for 24 hours after general anesthesia. If your operation is longer or more complicated—for example, if you have had a mastectomy with reconstruction—you may need to stay overnight in the hospital. In this case, you may be given the option of patient-controlled analgesia (PCA) for treating any postoperative pain. This is a syringe pump device that connects to your IV and is activated

BEFORE SURGERY: CONSULT WITH YOUR ANESTHESIOLOGIST

It is important to make certain that you understand what type of anesthesia you will receive and how it will affect you. Before surgery, ask your anesthesiologist:

- What type of anesthesia will I have?

- Will I be awake or asleep during my surgery?

- If I will be awake, how awake will I be?

- How will the anesthesia be administered?

- Will I have any tubes in my mouth or throat?

- How long will the effects of anesthesia last?

- Will I be nauseous? Is there any medication that I can receive while I'm asleep to prevent nausea?

- If you are on medication and you are asked not to eat or drink anything before surgery, is it okay to take your medication with a sip of water in the morning?

- If your surgery entails any type of sedation or general anesthesia, make sure to have someone drive you home from surgery.

when you push the button. It will deliver a preset dose of pain medication, such as Demerol or morphine, directly into your IV. You can decide when you get the medication, it takes effect immediately, and there is no shot. There will be limits placed so that you can't overdose yourself even if you push the button frequently.

You may also be given pneumatic stockings on your lower legs to help prevent blood clots during longer procedures. Pneumatic stockings are mechanical devices that intermittently inflate and deflate around your calf muscles to help keep your blood flowing. Generally you will be in them before surgery and until you are fully awake. Anytime you are kept immobile for significant periods of time without moving your legs there is an increased risk of blood clots developing in your legs, so you will wear them until you are up and walking. A blood clot in your legs could lead to pulmonary embolism in which a blood clot in a deep vein in your leg breaks loose and lodges in your lungs. This is a serious condition that requires being placed on blood thinner medication and occasionally having a mechanical filter placed in the vena cava (the major vein that leads to the heart).

While anesthesia does entail some risks, it has gotten much safer recently due to advances in technology and pharmacology. There are newer monitoring devices that greatly improve safety and newer anesthetic drugs and equipment that make anesthesia safer and better tolerated by patients than in the past. For example, capnography measures the carbon dioxide that you exhale when you are receiving ventilation and is used to make sure that the breathing tube is in the right spot. If you are having IV sedation, capnography can also be used as an apnea monitor to alert the anesthesiologist if you stop breathing.

Pulse oximetry measures the amount of oxygen in the bloodstream through a device that clips onto your finger. By measuring oxygen saturation, your anesthesiologist will get an early warning sign if something is wrong and can take corrective action.

Before surgery, your anesthesiologist will be able to answer many of your questions and help you decide which anesthetic technique is best for you. If you are extremely concerned about anesthesia or have significant medical problems, you can request a preoperative anesthesia consult to discuss your concerns with your anesthesiologist prior to the actual day of surgery. If you have diabetes, you may need to reduce your diabetic medications the evening before surgery in order to avoid a drop in your blood sugar on the morning of surgery. If you are on blood thinners, let your surgeon know at least one week prior to surgery so that arrangements can be made for the blood to clot normally during surgery.

CHAPTER FOURTEEN

Managing Recurrent
Breast Cancer

By John Barstis, M.D.

Most recurrences of breast cancer happen within the first five years of initial diagnosis, and the risk of having a recurrence decreases with time. However, recurrences can happen at any time, even after a woman has been disease-free for many years. Your risk of recurrence can be estimated from the information we have about the size of the primary tumor, the degree of lymph node involvement, and biological characteristics of the tumor tissue.

Without adjuvant therapy, the estimated lifetime risk of recurrence ranges from:

• Five percent for tumors of less than one centimeter, no nodal involvement, and all favorable tissue tests—for example, positive estrogen and progesterone receptors, and a negative her2/neu test.

• Twenty percent for a two- to three-centimeter, node-negative, estrogen receptor–negative cancer.

• Seventy to ninety percent when a five-centimeter tumor occurs with ten positive lymph nodes.

YOUR RISK OF RECURRENCE IS UNIQUE

The risk of recurrence is individualized. It's important to know that many people said to be at risk for recurrence never experience a recurrence. Adjuvant therapy, including chemotherapy and hormone therapy, can reduce the risk of recurrence significantly.

As discussed in Chapter 10, "Chemotherapy, Hormone Therapy, and the Stages of Breast Cancer," adjuvant therapy can dramatically lower this risk, in some cases more than 50 percent. It is extremely important to understand that the estimates of risk have limited value for any one individual and that many people said to be at high risk never experience a recurrence. Secondly, no one is without some risk of getting cancer but women who have had cancer are usually intensely aware of their cancer risk. People who have had cancer often overestimate their risk of getting cancer again and may be sensitive to life's other risks as well.

We categorize cancer recurrences according to the extent of their involvement. In so doing, we refer to local, regional, or systemic processes. The approach to each category of recurrence is different, so care must be taken when initially defining the extent of recurrence. Diagnosis, which is based on knowledge of the natural history of breast cancer and where it is likely to spread, is the first consideration.

Assessing the Possibility of a New Cancer

When new disease is suspected, we must consider tissue diagnosis. Only when the sum of all the initial evidence makes diagnosis of recurrence certain or nearly certain will a new biopsy be unnecessary. Otherwise, biopsy is needed to make sure that a recurrence has in fact taken place. A hot spot on a bone scan or a mass on a CT scan is not by itself proof of a recurrence. These occurrences can only be diagnostic within the proper clinical context. If you have an accessible abnormality, such as skin nodule, breast mass, or a lymph node, a fine needle aspiration, core needle biopsy, or excisional biopsy is indicated. In the hands of a skilled doctor, usually a surgeon or pathologist, a needle biopsy or excisional biopsy can help rule the presence of new cancer in or out.

A negative fine needle aspiration requires careful consultation to be sure that the actual tumor wasn't missed. An internal tumor may also be reached by fine needle aspiration or core needle biopsy, which employs a slightly thicker needle to get a more substantial specimen. A biopsy deep inside the body requires the use of a CT scan or ultrasound. In some cases, the location of a lesion may make these procedures technically difficult or somewhat risky, such as when the lesion is behind or adjacent to major blood vessels. Competent radiologists are often very skillful at making such judgments and can be trusted to guide you and your oncologist in such situations.

When tissue cannot be easily obtained, other tests might be of great value. These include the blood tests called *tumor markers*, most often CA15-3 or CA2729 for breast cancer. Essentially, these tests are diagnostic if the presence of cancer is markedly abnormal, although they can be misleading when only mildly elevated. MRI scans for certain types of tissue, such as brain, liver, or bone, can be nearly definitive. The PET (positron emission tomography) scan has become widely available. This is a functional scan that detects the abnormal metabolism of even the tiniest amount of tumor and is the most definitive noninvasive test yet developed for detection. However, it is very expensive and not always reliable outside of major medical centers.

The hardest thing is that you're so vulnerable. When you have a recurrence, it absolutely destroys your faith that this is going to end. You have to learn how to get that back or learn to live with it. • Joelle

If a Recurrence Is Detected

The next goal will be to establish the extent of recurrence. If local or regional recurrence is suspected, you will usually have a CT scan of your chest and abdomen and a bone scan. Depending on the clinical situation, other tests, such as an MRI scan of your head or a CT scan of your pelvis or of other sites, may also be appropriate.

Treating a Local Recurrence

If restaging shows that the recurrence is only in the breast, or after a mastectomy, on the chest wall, we can focus our attention solely upon that site. Systemic therapy is not usually given. If you have previously had breast-saving surgery—that is, wide excision, lumpectomy, or quadrantectomy—and radiotherapy, mastectomy is generally the best approach, with the most reconstructive options available to you.

> **DEFINING TYPES OF RECURRENCE**
>
> *Local recurrence* can be thought of as a recurrence in the breast or in the chest wall directly underneath the area where the breast was if you have had a mastectomy.
>
> *Regional recurrence* can be described as a recurrence in the chest wall (if you have not had a mastectomy) or the areas bordering the breast, including the axillary lymph nodes.
>
> *Systemic recurrence* is a recurrence in the distant organs.

If you have had a mastectomy, excision of the recurrence, when possible, and radiotherapy to the chest wall is the best option, if radiotherapy has not already been used. If you have had radiotherapy, you may not be able to have it again. Yet there are special techniques and approaches that may be available to you, such as microwave hyperthermia or small-field reirradiation, which is covered in Chapter 11, "Radiotherapy: What to Know, What to Ask."

The prognosis for a truly localized recurrence, including a recurrence that is confined to the breast or chest wall only, is generally very good with the exception of a very rapid local recurrence, which has a more guarded prognosis.

Treating a Regional Recurrence

A regional recurrence is when all restaging tests show that the cancer has returned to the soft tissues or nodes bordering the breast. This includes the chest wall bordering the breast area and the supraclavicular region (the region just above the clavicle). Radiation therapy and possibly surgery (but this is less likely) is the recommended treatment in this setting. If a recurrence develops in the axilla (armpit), the approach will be very individualized, as surgery to remove lymph nodes has usually already been done and arm swelling is a risk. If surgery to remove the recurrence can be performed safely, it should be done. Systemic therapy may also be considered. Although there is no clear approach to systemic therapy in this situation, chemotherapy may be considered if it has not been previously given, and hormonal therapy may be given if the cancer receptor is positive.

> **WHEN YOU HAVE A RECURRENCE**
>
> If you have a recurrence you can feel, see your surgical oncologist.
>
> If a recurrence is identified on an X ray or blood test, see your medical oncologist for advice.
>
> It is always a good idea to see a doctor on your original team, as he or she will have first-hand knowledge about your medical history and treatment.

Systemic Recurrence

Breast cancer that recurs in any area beyond those we've just discussed is presumed to have traveled through the bloodstream, making any other area of the body, such as the bones, liver, lungs, and brain, at risk for recurrence. Any distant metastasis is serious and usually considered incurable. Yet, the expected survival rate after recurrence is highly variable and is often many years long due to increasingly effective therapies. If you have no treatment or treatment does not lengthen your survival time, survival may be no longer than six to twelve months once metastatic disease is diagnosed in the liver.

Despite the term, soft tissue includes bones as well as the body's connective tissues. (*Soft tissue* can be defined as any supporting structure of the body that is not an organ.) A person with metastatic disease in the soft tissues only would be estimated to have a chance of survival of one to two years, if not treated or the treatment is unsuccessful.

When your overall condition (called *performance status*) is good, meaning that the effects of the cancer and any coexisting medical problems have not significantly impaired your body's functions, an aggressive approach to maximizing survival is undertaken. The younger a woman is, and the more limited the amount of recurrence, the more likely an aggressive approach is to be taken. Thus, one or two isolated recurrences, even if in the lung or liver, may warrant consideration for removal in certain cases. Radiation may be considered the first intervention in an area of soft tissue or bone and is routinely given if this area is painful or symptomatic in some other way. In most cases, systemic therapy is given, but the approach varies greatly depending on many factors. Hormone and chemotherapy are the two major types of systemic therapy.

Treating Recurrence with Hormone Therapy

Hormone therapy is an option when tumor tissue is found to be either estrogen or progesterone receptor positive, or both. If the original breast primary tumor was positive, the metastases are usually presumed to be as well. Tamoxifen (Novladex) is the prototypical hormone medication. It functions as an antiestrogen on breast cancer cells and can potentially bring about long-lasting remissions, often with minimal or no side effects. There are more than half-a-dozen new agents that have been developed as improvements on the tamoxifen model. Early studies have demonstrated their superiority to tamoxifen in many cases. The largest group of these agents is called *aromatase inhibitors.* The FDA has approved several of these agents, including letrozole (the trade name is Femara) and anastrozole (Arimidex). Like tamoxifen, they are in pill form and, like tamoxifen, they are best used in situations that are not immediately life-threatening, such as in soft tissue disease, because they can take up to one to two months to achieve full efficacy. They can provide remission of cancer that can last from several months to several years and occasionally longer, and when one agent fails, another can be substituted.

Chemotherapy in Recurrent Breast Cancer

When disease is critical or progressing readily, chemotherapy is often the best treatment. Chapter 10, "Chemotherapy, Hormone Therapy, and the Stages of Breast Cancer," explains the many different agents that are available, some of which were developed quite recently. They cannot cure metastatic disease, but they can often bring about substantial improvement in the disease with fewer side effects than with medications used in the past. This includes complete remissions in some patients, which may last many years. It is beyond the scope of this chapter to try to list all of the agents and combinations in use for metastatic breast cancer. As with adjuvant therapy, the most effective available agents are Adriamycin and the taxanes, Taxotere and Taxol. We can use these agents by themselves or in combination with others, depending on the level of intensity deemed appropriate for the situation. Gemcitabine, vinorelbine, and capcitabene are among other new effective agents.

Entirely new treatments are now in development, and a few are available or are very close to approval at the time of this writing. The best-known example at present is Herceptin, an antibody or immune treatment aimed at a protein present in excessive amounts on the surface of the cell, when there is a change inside the cell called her-2 overexpression. Between 10 to 20 percent of breast cancers have this defect and can be treated with Herceptin. In such cases, Herceptin can dramatically improve a woman's survival. Other agents called *angiogenesis inhibitors* and *tyrosine kinase inhibitors* are in clinical trials at the time of this writing and will clearly be useful options in the battle against breast cancer. A woman with breast cancer who wants to fight her disease aggressively should always be sure that she learns what clinical trials may be available to her. Clinical trials are now a core part of the care of breast cancer. (The resource directory at the end of this book lists several sources of further information about clinical trials.)

Treating Pain and Discomfort: Palliative Therapy

When a woman decides that she wishes efforts to be directed at her comfort, more than toward prolonging her life, the focus shifts to using interventions that can provide immediate benefit. Comfort therapy (also called *palliative therapy*) usually focuses on the treatment of symptoms such as pain, nausea, weakness, lack of appetite, and depression.

Pain is the most obvious problem that palliative efforts must address. Almost always, we must perform tests to ascertain the cause of the pain. For example, severe pain in an extremity might be due to a spontaneous fracture from a metastasis, called a *pathologic fracture*. This can be rapidly remedied by an internal pinning orthopedic surgical procedure. A simple bone X ray of a painful area may prove very valuable and, in some cases, MRI may prove more definitive. In other cases, pain may come from swelling or irritation of an organ by a metastasis, such as in the liver. In these situations, pain medication alone is less effective than specific targeted remedies.

If the sources of pain are multiple and preclude these types of therapy, we then focus primarily on the optimal use of pain medications. Currently the most frequently used model is the World Health Organization three-step ladder approach. The first rung on the ladder consists of:

- Nonopioid analgesics such as acetominophen.

- Nonsteroidal anti-inflammatory agents such as ibuprofen, naprosyn, celebrex, and vioxx.

These medications all have daily maximums that should not be exceeded for more than a very short time, as they can be toxic to the liver and kidneys.

The next rung on the ladder adds:

- Mild opioids such as hydrocodone or codeine that are sold mixed with acetominophen. These include the trade names Vicodin, Lorcet, and Norco.

The third step consists of:

- Stronger opioids such as oxycodone, dilaudid, and morphine. Meperidine, or Demerol, is also on the list, but it is not a good choice as its first breakdown product of the body is toxic to the nervous system, although Demerol can be safely used for treating acute or short-term pain. The first three agents in this list have no upper limits in dose and can be gradually increased as much as necessary to achieve comfort. Morphine and Oxycodone are both available as long-acting preparations. There is also Duragesic, a long-acting patch worn on the skin. Doctors or nurses who are familiar with the special characteristics of these drugs should supervise all of the long-acting medications.

The Estrogen Dilemma and Breast Cancer

By Maurice Cohen, M.D., F.A.C.S., F.A.C.O.G., F.A.C.E.

The changes that young women experience at puberty, changes that result in the majesty of the female body and mind, are due to the introduction of the ovarian hormones estrogen and progesterone into the body. These hormones stimulate breast tissue, develop the shape and contour of your breasts, awaken the menstrual cycle, ignite your sex drive, and make it possible to give birth. But while estrogen, in particular, is a tremendous contributor to your emotional and sexual life, and to your vitality and creativity, it is also associated with your risk of breast cancer.

Estrogen is actually a group of hormones that travel to every cell in the body, where they are capable of altering cellular function, resulting in changes that vary according to the estrogen receptors that are present in the cell as well as the type of receptor that predominates in the cell. We now know that cells can have both alpha and beta estrogen receptors and that they vary in amount and quality in different organ systems.

During your lifetime, you are exposed to estrogens within your own body as well as from without—for example, if you eat a diet that contains small amounts of estrogen, if you are exposed to environmental contaminants with estrogenic activity, or if you take estrogen hormones. Although we don't clearly understand why, the risk of developing breast cancer is lower when estrogen is not present. We do know that risk factors for breast cancer include:

- Beginning menstruation before the age of 12.

- Late menopause—that is, after the age of 55

- Having your first pregnancy after 30 or no pregnancy

- Not breast-feeding

Women who have a slightly elevated bone density also seem to have a higher risk of breast cancer, probably because the more than ample amount of estrogen they are exposed to creates stronger bones and at the same time has negative effects on breast tissue. We also see the risk of breast cancer increase with women who produce excessive amounts of estrogen without progesterone due to a condition known as *polycystic ovarian syndrome*. These women have a higher risk of breast and uterine cancer. Too much estrogen can also cause breast pain, swelling, and detectable changes on a routine mammogram.

Many strategies used to treat breast cancer include drugs that block the estrogen receptor in breast cells, such as tamoxifen and raloxifene. Aromatase inhibitors, used to treat metastatic breast cancer, work by blocking the conversion of androgens to estrogens in peripheral fat tissue. If you are overweight or have a hip-to-waist ratio that is associated with visceral fat (that is, the classic "apple" shape, in which you store more fat in your stomach than elsewhere), you are also at greater risk because estrogen can be peripherally produced and stored in fat and stomach fat is more biologically active than other types of fat. We also know that leading a sedentary life puts women at risk and that increased fiber intake and exercise may decrease the risk. Estrogen and progesterone play a significant role in a woman's body, but the levels and type of hormones can be modified. If you are being treated for breast cancer, your breast cancer team, including your surgical oncologist and medical oncologist, are your first line of defense in battling the disease. Be sure to discuss any of the concepts in this chapter with your physician before putting them into practice.

Hormone Replacement Therapy (HRT)

For more than 35 years, women experience the production of estrogens orchestrated by the pituitary hormones, along with ovulation and the addition of progesterone to the second half of the menstrual cycle until perimenopause when the ovary begins a subtle but steady decline in function. Ultimately one loses the ability to ovulate, to produce progesterone, and then to produce estrogens. The final menstrual period signals that the ovaries no longer function as they used to. When this happens, changes can be noted in every body system. Because your body has responded to its own ovarian milieu for decades, it's not surprising that the changes leading to the end of ovarian function are associated with difficult mind/body symptoms.

Yet, there is a wide spectrum of menopausal symptoms. Some women have no symptoms at all, some have symptoms that subside with time, and others, at the opposite end of the spectrum, are encumbered by symptoms so severe that they can only be relieved by ovarian hormone replacement. It's not uncommon for women approaching menopause to experience:

- Sleep disturbance

- Changes in body heat, such as hot flashes

- Changes in vaginal wetness

- Mood changes

- Changes in the ability to handle personal and work-related stress

- Changes in creative energy

- Changes in cognitive function and the ability to concentrate and focus

- Decline in sexual interest or responsiveness

While the age of the final menstrual period has not changed with time, our life expectancy has changed. At the turn of the century, a woman's life expectancy corresponded to the final menstrual period. Medical advances and improvements in our physical environment have increased our life expectancy appreciably, so that a woman entering the twenty-first century can expect to live at least a third of her life after the end of her ovarian function. The advent of the women's movement and the birth control pill brought many women into the workforce with opportunities far different from those of their mothers and grandmothers and with very different expectations. Today, maintaining ongoing effectiveness and vitality during and after menopause are topics of importance to women, especially to women who maintain a high level of professional and personal activity. Many choose to treat the hormone alteration of the menopause with hormone replacement therapy (HRT), replenishing hormones that have declined.

The Advent of Hormone Replacement Therapy

In 1966, Robert Wilson, M.D., a gynecologist practicing at Methodist Hospital in Brooklyn, New York, attracted the public's attention when he wrote about the consequences of hormonal changes in menopause in his book *Forever Feminine.* Although roundly criticized by the profession, the book was a best-seller and set a trend for using hormone replacement therapy to maintain vitality that still continues today.

Because of the obvious benefits to health, ongoing vitality, and longevity, hormone replacement therapy has become a mainstream choice for many. Most women today take hormone replacement therapy to address some of the effects of menopause. Yet misconceptions about hormone replacement therapy remain, especially with regard to beneficial effects on osteoporosis and cardiovascular health.

While estrogen has a favorable effect on lipids and blood vessels, the notion that estrogen provides an adequate means of preventing heart disease is misleading. A woman who is overweight, for example, or who smokes, has elevated blood pressure, or has high cholesterol will require individualized strategies to address these issues. If you have heart disease, a good cardiologist can advise you of an overall health plan that's right for you. Similarly, there are many effective medications to treat osteoporosis. You may not need hormone replacement therapy, but you may need medication, calcium, vitamin D, and exercise. If, however, you are taking estrogen to address quality-of-life issues, and you do in fact need hormones for that reason, you will get the added benefit of bone stabilization, but, again, you don't generally need estrogen solely for this purpose.

Does Estrogen Replacement Affect the Risk of Breast Cancer?

Epidemiologists offer two different points of view on this question. The first, popularized by the late Trudy Bush from the University of Maryland, is that the studies do not slow a clear positive relationship. If there is a relationship, it's small and doesn't outweigh the tremendous benefits gained by the replacement of ovarian hormones. The other point of view is that the long-term replacement does alter the risk of developing breast cancer, and that the risk is proportional to the amount and the duration of exposure. All agree that short-term use—that is, less than five years—of conventional hormone replacement to control symptoms poses little risk.

We believe that the solution to solving problems related to estrogen lies in encouraging strategies that will modify estrogen activity in the body and enhance safety. These include proper diet, exercise, stress management and emotional support, maintaining liver and intestinal health, eliminating toxins from your body, and increasing your intake of sources of antioxidants and phytoestrogens, which are plant-based estrogens that can be found in whole foods like soy. When severe menopausal symptoms necessitate treatment, there are safer nonhormonal methods as well as short-term low-dose hormonal strategies available for most women with breast cancer, women who are at risk, and women who don't want to take hormones.

Natural Approaches to Hormone Therapy

The first estrogens available for clinical use over 50 years ago were the estrogenic substances extracted from the urine of pregnant mares called *conjugated equine estrogens (CEE)*, brand name Premarin, Premarin contains substances that are structurally similar to human estrogens along with hormones characteristic of the horse. Premarin represented a major breakthrough and is widely used today, being an effective therapeutic agent, one that is still considered the gold standard. Most women using hormone replacement therapy report satisfaction with CEE.

As mentioned earlier, the human ovary produces different types of estrogen, including estrone (E1), 17-beta-estradiol (E2), and estriol (E3), all of which have been isolated and are available from plant sources for clinical use. These plant-derived estrogens are referred to as *natural* or *bioidentical estrogens.* The production of hormones from plant sources is based on the work of chemist Russell E. Marker who first derived progesterone from the Mexican yam in the 1940s. Because hormone deficiency involves the absence of these estrogens, there is growing agreement among clinicians that HRT should involve the use of these bioidentical hormones rather than the equine-based mixtures. The bioidentical hormones are species-specific to the human, rather than species-specific to the horse, as is the case with equilins. Further, there is now evidence that some of the liver's metabolic effects of these equilins are different than the metabolites of the bioidentical estrogens. Plant-derived hormones are structurally similar to the hormones women produce themselves and they metabolize in the same way as women's natural hormones. This is the reason for the growing sentiment among clinicians that these hormones may be safer than the equilin-derived hormones.

The question of hormone replacement therapy use is even further complicated by the addition of synthetic progesterone, called *progestin*, to traditional hormone replacement regimens. Two recent studies on HRT and breast cancer have shown that the risk of breast cancer increases when estrogens are used with progestins instead of estrogen-only therapies. But plant-derived progesterone is available for use. This bioidentical, natural progesterone is not as strong as the synthetics and therefore maybe safer. The hard scientific conclusions are not in yet, but these estrogens from plant sources may provide a margin of safety over equilin compounds. The dosages must be tailored to the needs of the patient and changed with prolonged use. I believe that the one-size-fits-all strategy for hormone replacement must be seriously challenged. Giving the same dose of HRT to a 50-year-old woman with severe menopausal symptoms as well as to an 80-year-old woman whose needs involve Alzheimer's prevention and quality-of-life issues violates basic pharmaceutical principles and should be discouraged.

The "Good" and the "Bad" Estrogens

H. Leon Bradlow, Ph.D., the emeritus director of the Biochemical Endocrinology Lab at the Strang Cancer Research Laboratory at New York University, talks about "good" and "bad" estrogens in his work. Estrogens produced in the ovaries are metabolized into two major groups, the C-2 and C-16. The good estrogens are metabolites with C-2 structure, and the bad are the C-16 metabolites. C-2 compounds appear less strong than the C-16 compounds and seem to be associated with a decreased incidence of breast and uterine cancer. Bradlow contends that the ratio between the two can be influenced by exercise and by eating cruciferous vegetables like broccoli, cauliflower, kale, brussel sprouts, turnips, rutabaga, and cabbage. The cruciferous vegetables all have a phytochemical called *indole-3-carbinol (I3C)*. Many of the beneficial effects of isoflavones found in soy, for example, are also due to indole-3-carbinol. In his book *Frontiers Two*, published in 1993, Isaac Asimov notes that, "Chemicals in cruciferous vegetables, like cabbage and broccoli, lower the risk of breast cancer by increasing the metabolism of estrogen, breaking it down to an inactive form."

A few salient questions come to mind when we look at synthetic hormones versus those that are plant-derived: Are those estrogens that have dominated clinical use more potent and do they have more potential for stimulating the breast excessively, thus increasing the risk of breast cancer? Can the stimulation to the breast tissue be decreased by the use of soy products, vegetables, and plant-derived estrogens? If we can influence the safety of estrogen nutritionally, as Bradlow has shown, then would it be reasonable to expect that a weaker estrogen that has been metabolized by human beings for millions of years is safer than synthetic or conjugated hormones that are not involved in the natural evolutionary biodegradable process? I believe that the metabolic processes of degrading bioidentical hormones are different and probably safer than the synthetic or conjugated hormones.

The Women's Health Initiative (WHI) sponsored by the National Institutes of Health is the largest clinical trial investigating factors that affect women's health and longevity, with 162,000 women recruited into the study at a cost of $625 million. The effects of CEE and Provera, synthetic progesterone given in some hormone replacement therapy regimens, are being studied. Regretfully, the effect of hormone replacement using bioidentical hormones is not included in the study. If the plant-derived estrogen and progesterone are indeed safer to use than CEE and progestins, the answer will not be forthcoming from the WHI effort.

Hormone Replacement Therapy and Cancer Risk

There are times during the perimenopausal stage of life— that is, before the final menstrual period—when a woman has symptoms for which she desires relief. The judicious, short-term use of birth control pills, low-dose estrogens, and natural progesterone cream in appropriate dosage and time of cycle can be helpful. But the use of these methods must be individualized, considering the degree of symptoms and each person's risk of breast cancer. For example, if you are at risk for breast cancer and have severe menopausal symptoms, you might opt for short-term use of birth control pills or low-dose natural hormones to address severe symptoms immediately while beginning to use nonhormonal strategies, which, while effective, take time to work. By using nonhormonal strategies, such as diet and exercise, you will be facilitating future choices for short- or long-term use of hormones. If you opt for short-term use under these circumstances, discontinuation will not cause a rebound of symptoms.

If you have a family history of breast cancer, biopsies that are atypical, or you don't want to use hormones, yet you have symptoms of menopause for which you need relief, there are other options. Bellergal S, an old formulation of autonomic nervous system stabilizers, or clonidine, an antihypertensive agent, can be used. Low-dose antidepressants may also be helpful. Some herbs, such as black cohosh root, can be useful for menopausal symptoms, although they may take some time to work. Vaginal dryness can be treated with vitamin E suppositories, vitamin E

| IS ESTROGEN SAFE FOR YOU?

Estrogen is safe for most women; however, there are some patients for whom there is probably some risk of breast cancer development with estrogen. As long as these patients know the risks, have discussed them with their doctors, and understand the possible ramifications, they can take estrogen if they need it. These include:

• Patients who have had Stage 1 breast cancer but who have been cancer-free for five years.

• Patients with first-generation relatives who have had breast cancer, including a mother, sister, or daughter.

• Patients who have had atypia or LCIS (lobular carcinoma in situ) diagnosed on prior breast biopsies.

• Patients who have had ductal carcinoma in situ (DCIS) on a prior breast biopsy.

There is a group of patients for whom estrogen is generally contraindicated. These patients include:

• Patients who, within the last five years, have had a diagnosis of breast cancer, especially if it is estrogen or progesterone receptor positive.

• Patients with metastatic breast cancer.

• Patients who are being treated with tamoxifen.

• Patients who are BRCA 1 or BRCA 2 positive.

There are, however, exceptions to these recommendations, and each patient must consult her own specialist to make these decisions.

cream in a neutral base, and/or the topical use of pure vitamin E oil. There are other lubricants, like Astroglide, Replens, or K-Y jelly, but they have a less favorable effect on the mucosa (the mucous membrane of the vagina). If you have breast cancer, or are at an increased risk for breast cancer, and vitamin E preparations have not worked for you, you can use some topical estrogens in low doses. The local use of Estriol cream in low concentrations is effective on vaginal tissue, but has little or no systemic effect and will not affect risk. (There is some thinking that estriol is protective against breast cancer.) Estriol cream is available from formulating pharmacies (special pharmacies that compound formulations to order). Its use should be encouraged as a reasonable and safe treatment for this common problem. Most doctors, including gynecologists, who are interested in menopausal medicine and in bioidentical hormones, work with formulating pharmacies around the country and can write a prescription for you, if you have special needs.

If you have breast cancer, it's especially important that you receive individualized treatment, information, support, and care. This is particularly true if you have not reached menopause by the time of your diagnosis. Chemotherapy can suppress ovarian function and cause early menopause with symptoms that are more severe than with menopause that is gradual and spontaneous. For most women, the nonhormonal strategies of diet, exercise, and the addition of isoflavones, bioflavonoids, antioxidants, and stress management alleviate the need for hormone replacement. But there are times when quality-of-life issues necessitate the use of hormone replacement. In these rare instances when other strategies, such as herbal preparations, diet changes, and antidepressants have not worked, low-dose natural estrogens and the use of natural progesterone from plant sources can be recommended. If you are interested in the possibility of using low-dose natural estrogens, tell your doctor that you do not want synthetic progesterone and that you only want estrogens that are identical to the estrogens in your body. While it is controversial, there are some who feel that the addition of estriol enhances anti-cancer activity, and that Tri-Estrogen, which contains estriol, estradiol, and estrone, should be one of the choices given to women who have tried and not succeeded with other strategies. Megace is a progestin that is used to treat metastatic uterine and breast cancer. In low doses, Megace can be used to treat hot flashes that are unresponsive to other strategies.

When these hormones are used, every effort should be made to begin using nonhormonal strategies as soon as possible so that hormone exposure can be time-limited and kept low with regard to dosage. It is important to realize that hormones can be but a bridge to other strategies that can empower you to take control over the way you feel. For example, you might want to investigate yoga, meditation, support groups, or other useful practices. It is clear that menopausal transition for women with breast cancer or women at high risk for developing breast cancer require a team approach, involving the surgeon, oncologist, and gynecologist, along with nutritionists and holistic practitioners who deal with nutritional and stress-reduction strategies. The more input you have from those who are treating you, the more likely you are to maintain your quality of life during this difficult time.

CHAPTER SIXTEEN

New Approaches to Breast Health: Understanding Complementary Medicine

By Steven M. Rosman, Ph.D., L.A.c., M.S., D.A.P.A.

More than two hundred years ago, Percival Pott, M.D., a London physician, described scrotal cancers in men who had worked as chimney sweeps in their youth. Pott's description represented one of the first pieces of medical documentation to explain cancer as a result of lifestyle and environmental factors. Since then, researchers have noted increased cases of specific cancers among miners in eastern Germany, X-ray technicians, women who painted luminescent radium on the hands of wristwatches, and cigarette smokers. Clearly, the opinion that one's lifestyle and environment play a role in cancer development is no longer a lonely one.

Complementary medicine, also referred to as integrative or holistic medicine, takes an individual's lifestyle and environment into account when making treatment recommendations. Complementary medicine's perspective is represented by the American Holistic Health Association's statement: "Rather than focusing on illness or specific parts of the body, holistic health considers the whole person and how it interacts with its environment. It emphasizes the connection of body, mind, and spirit. Holistic health is based on the law of nature that a whole is made of interdependent parts. The earth is made up of systems, such as air, land, water, plants, and animals. If life is to be sustained, they cannot be separated, for what is happening to one is also felt by all the other systems. In the same way, an individual is a whole made up of interdependent parts, which are the physical, mental, emotional, and spiritual. When one part is not working at its best, it will impact all the other parts of that person."

From the perspective of a practitioner of complementary medicine, breast health is maintained through proper diet, appropriate nutritional supplementation, exercise, stress management, and avoiding environmental toxins, as well as cultivating an optimism and a passion for life. Medical research supports complementary approaches, as Dr. Frederica Perera's statement in the prestigious medical journal *Science* (May 1996) exemplifies: "The likelihood of tumor development is increased by impairment of the immune system and by such disorders as hormonal imbalances, hepatitis, and chronic lung disease. Convincing evidence also indicates that a diet low in fruits and vegetables containing antioxidants and other nutrients (such as vitamins A, C, and E) increases the probability of acquiring diverse cancers . . . the effect of any one, single-acting gene can be modulated by environmental influences, by other genes, by health and nutritional status, and by an array of other host characteristics." Indeed, some medical researchers believe that if genetic vulnerability may account for about 18,000 new cases of cancer annually, the environment may account for more than 160,000. Genes do not necessarily dictate outcome.

We know that the genes BRCA-1 and BRCA-2 are implicated in the initiation and development of breast cancer. When they function normally, they act as tumor suppressor genes that help regulate healthy cell division. But when these genes malfunction, cells within specific tissues can proliferate and give rise to tumors in the breast, colon, brain, skin, or lungs. We cannot assume, however, that the identification of these genes in an individual is a tragic portent of cancer. A growing number of researchers are beginning to echo Dr. Perera's words. Consider for example, what Jeffrey Bland, Ph.D., says in his book *Genetic Nutritioneering:* "Investigators from a number of scientific and medical disciplines are discovering that it is not just the genes that influence risk of cancer. Much of the risk depends on the modification in expression of those genes through diet, lifestyle, and environmental factors.

Although we do not presently have the technology to modify our genes, we certainly can modify our diet, lifestyle, and environmental exposures once we have been informed of our specific risks."

"The Couch Potato Syndrome" and Other Lifestyle Factors That Influence Breast Cancer Risk

In his study of 90,000 nurses over four years, Dr. Walter Willet of the Harvard School of Public Health found that among other things the nurses who consumed zero to two drinks of alcohol a week had no increased risk of breast cancer while those who consumed three to nine drinks a week elevated their risk by 30 percent. Young women appear to be the most affected. Although drinking at any age should not be encouraged, those with increased risk factors for breast cancer should limit any alcoholic beverages.

The well-known couch potato syndrome, or sedentary lifestyle, is another risk factor for breast cancer. Exercising before menopause can reduce the exposure breast cells have to hormones that could promote cancer. Indeed, research conducted with more than a thousand women at the University of Southern California's North Cancer Center found that moderate exercise done at least three to four hours per week can alter monthly exposure to excess estrogen. However, it is this author's experience that moderate exercise ought to be done daily in some form. Do what gives you pleasure. Take a walk after dinner, dance, swim, play hopscotch, take the stairs rather than the escalator when you can— whatever makes you feel more active. We're not talking about aerobic fitness at this point. The idea is to get more oxygen into your system and to see yourself as active rather than ailing. You can start with small steps, and when you are ready, graduate to increased activity. But again, let your exercise be pleasurable and not simply another source of stress. Find what it is that you like to do, and pursue it.

Exercise is important even after menopause, because it can reduce body fat and result in a reduction of estrogen produced in fat tissue. These conclusions are supported by studies like the one in which the effects of exercise on 25,000 Norwegian women were observed and assessed. The authors of this study concluded that those who exercised at least four hours per week had a 37 percent lower risk of developing breast cancer.

Among other health benefits, regular exercise delays the onset of the first menstruation, thus reducing lifelong hormonal exposure. Regular exercise prevents the accumulation of excess body fat and those adipose (fat) cells wherein supplemental, unwanted estrogen can be produced. It also helps to diminish excess insulin production. As we shall see later, this is yet another reason exercise should be added to your breast health regimen.

Controlling Stress

I think as women we really need to look at how we're caring for ourselves. I had to realize that I was a perfectionist. Now I don't try to be "supermom." I learned that if it isn't perfect, it's all right. Meditation really helped me to be stress-free. • Joan

Stress is hard to define, but easy to spot. We know what distresses us, but we don't always know the effect it has on our bodies. While many of us will just grin and bear it, toughing it out has dire consequences for our health.

Stress is a part of our lives. We have all experienced it in one form or another. Illness is certainly very stressful. We can also be distressed by work, family pressures, relocations, injury, or the death of a loved one. Retirement, money problems, and school are also sources of stress. Even positive life events, such as moving or starting a new job, can cause stress, depending on our perception of the event. How do we know we are distressed? Well, we may notice:

- Rapid heartbeat
- Cold, clammy hands
- Trouble sleeping
- Constipation or loose bowels
- Backache
- Muscle aches
- Headaches
- Shortness of breath
- Indigestion
- Decreased appetite or craving unhealthy foods

- Chest pains or joint pains
- Numbness
- Fatigue

- No zest for life
- Melancholy
- Excessive crying

What's Wrong with Stress?

When we become distressed, our bodies respond by releasing hormones that send messages to organs and glands around the body causing biological changes that include increased heart rate, reduced digestive juices, increased shallow breathing, increased blood sugar levels, reduced power and number of important immune cells, breakdown of protein structures, injury to brain cells, loss of vital substances like electrolytes, exhaustion of adrenal glands, reduced blood circulation in some internal organs, and more. According to the medical literature, if these unhealthy physiological responses are allowed to continue over days, weeks, months, even years, they can contribute to:

- Angina (cardiac pain) and cardiovascular disease
- Anxiety and panic
- Asthma
- Autoimmune diseases like rheumatoid arthritis and lupus
- Cancers of all kinds
- Chronic pain
- Common cold

- Depression
- Adult onset diabetes
- Headaches of all kinds
- Hypertension (high blood pressure)
- Immune suppression
- Irritable bowel syndrome
- Menstrual irregularities
- Premenstrual tension syndrome
- Ulcerative colitis

Stress can deplete the body of nutrients that include a host of B vitamins, vitamin C, magnesium, and zinc. These nutrients help in the healthy metabolism of estrogen, keep the immune system strong and watchful against mutations and unwanted cell growth, and help maintain adrenal glands. Stress can alter the balance of healthy and unhealthy intestinal flora, which, as we shall see, helps to convert certain plant foods into important estrogen modulators and helps to reduce levels of a bacterial enzyme that can increase the reabsorption of unwanted estrogen compounds.

Bouts of acute stress also diminish levels of circulating natural killer cells. These cells play a vital role in immune system surveillance against viruses and cancer cells. Repeated bouts of acute stress that become chronic stressors to our system debilitate our capacity to defend against serious health threats like cancer. A review article in the prestigious *American Journal of Surgery* (1995) concluded that relaxation, guided imagery, hypnosis, and other relaxation techniques boosted and balanced critical immune functions. With this in mind, I advise you to seek out stress-management programs in your community that offer the kind of strategies that appeal to you. Successful stress management strategies might include yoga, meditation, chi gong, tai chi, humor, exercise, cognitive therapy, breath work, autogenic training (a way to achieve a relaxed state), aromatherapy, and music, among others. You can find information about these stress management techniques from a variety of sources. For example, most psychologists and people trained in social work are familiar with autogenic training. Those steeped in ancient healing traditions, such as chi gong and tai chi, should be familiar with breath work. Your doctor's office, Yellow Pages, community center, or health club might also be able to offer information about classes and services in your area.

Social Support Affects Breast Health

Loneliness and isolation increase the risk of suboptimal breast health. Groundbreaking research published in 1989 by Stanford University psychiatrist David Spiegel, M.D., convincingly demonstrated that social support helps to prolong lives of women with breast cancer. It's now well-known that Dr. Spiegel initially wanted to debunk claims that mind-body techniques and social support might help cancer patients survive. So imagine his surprise when after ten years of study, Spiegel and his colleagues discovered that not only did women in his groups cope more effectively with their illnesses, they also lived twice as long as those who did not participate in groups.

Every person going through this (cancer diagnosis and treatment) should have someone they can draw alongside them, someone to listen and to be a source of support. I'm blessed with a wonderful husband. I didn't have to ask him to help me; he was there, and my children were there for me. But support groups are great. When I first found out that there was a possibility of cancer, I called a support person on the phone. She was able to direct me to the American Cancer Society, which can provide a lot of literature to help people on their journey. • Linda L.

A support group is really important. You can talk to other people with cancer, and caregivers can get information. Cancer can be traumatic for everyone who cares about the person with the disease. It has an effect on the children and the spouse of the person with the cancer. The whole family needs support. • Joelle

Most women like to talk things out. I recommend that women find a support group immediately. In support groups, you are in camaraderie with other women, and you can ask questions and share information. You get little tips; you feel like you belong. We would take our hats off at meetings, and we would all sit there with our little bald heads. You feel very accepted. I love the women I met at my support group. They are very important to me. • Anne

Several years later, another psychiatrist Dr. Fawzy I. Fawzy, this time at UCLA, discovered that patients who were most distressed at the beginning of his six-year study but who developed an active way of coping with their stress were significantly more likely to remain free of the disease. Like Spiegel, Fawzy conducted support groups for his patients to attend. His group sessions included various forms of therapy, such as cognitive strategies, relaxation techniques, and social interaction.

About the time Dr. Spiegel was publishing the results of his work with support groups, James House, Ph.D., of the University of Michigan, published his own review of a half-dozen studies of more than 22,000 men and women, where he found that people's social relationships or lack thereof constituted a major risk factor for ill health rivaling the effects of cigarette smoking, high blood pressure, obesity, and lack of physical activity.

The Power of Soy and Other Plant Foods

Breast cancer can be a hormonally driven tumor. That's why reducing the effect of the hormone most responsible for spurring the development and growth of the tumor is vital. Estrogen directly affects special cells called *epithelial cells* that line the inner surfaces of the breast's most susceptible tissues by causing the cells to divide excessively. Drugs like tamoxifen and raloxifene work by denying estrogen access to the receptors on those sensitive cells. Tamoxifen has been used in the treatment of breast cancer for over 25 years, and numerous studies have shown that it reduces the rate of breast cancer recurrence. In 1988, the FDA approved tamoxifen for patients at risk for the disease, where a 50 percent reduction rate was demonstrated. Although tamoxifen has an antiestrogenic affect on the breast receptor, it seems to have an estrogen-stimulating effect on the lining of the uterus, increasing the risk of endometrial polypi and endometrial cancer. There is also a concern that the estrogen receptor in the breast may alter its receptivity to tamoxifen after five years, becoming a stimulating agent to the receptor. Because of this possibility, tamoxifen use after five years is generally discouraged.

Raloxifene (Evista) is a SERM (selective estrogen receptor modulator) with FDA approval for the treatment and prevention of osteoporosis. (SERMs block the estrogen receptor on the surface of the cell. See chapter 10, "Chemotherapy, Hormone Therapy, and the Stages of Breast Cancer," for more information.) Like tamoxifen, raloxifene has a favorable effect on lipid profiles (cholesterol), although reduced incidences of coronary events like heart attack have not been shown. However, prospective studies have shown that raloxifene has breast cancer prevention activity similar to tamoxifen without the stimulating effect on the uterus. At the time of this writing, its breast cancer prevention effect has been observed for almost five years and there is consensus that it will be maintained and that the FDA will grant approval for this indication in the not-too-distant future. In the meantime, many clinicians are jumping the gun and using raloxifene as a breast cancer prevention agent along with its approved bone density feature.

Both tamoxifen and raloxifene increase hot flashes, and women often discontinue their use due to these troublesome symptoms. The problem seems to occur especially in women who are in their transitional years: either early perimenopause or early menopause, with the SERM exaggerating the natural symptoms. Using isoflavones, such as those found in soy (see below), and stress reduction techniques for several months before using a SERM seem to help to reduce hot flashes. Both tamoxifen and raloxifene are associated with a slight increased risk of blood clots in the legs, similar to those seen in estrogen users, and leg cramps. Women taking tamoxifen show an increased risk of depression, which may also apply to raloxifene users. Seventy percent of women taking tamoxifen report memory problems. Again, the data is not clear with raloxifene. Further SERM development holds out the possibility of having agents that are breast cancer protective, cardioprotective, and osteoporosis protective, and have a favorable effect on brain function and avoidance of hot flashes.

Some foods called *phytoestrogens*, or plant estrogens, block access to estrogen receptors, as does tamoxifen, but without the potential unwanted side effects. Most experts agree that increasing intake of soy products, such as tofu, among premenopausal women decreases the risk of several types of female cancers, particularly breast cancer. Soy products reduce the circulating levels of estradiol, the most active form of estrogen, because the phytoestrogens compete with estradiol for the binding of estrogen receptor sites. Because the phytoestrogens are weaker, they increase levels of sex hormone–binding globulin (SHBG), a carrier protein manufactured in the liver that transports estrogen, progesterone, and testosterone through the bloodstream to provide a reservoir of hormones ready for release as free or active hormones. This means that more estrogen might circulate in an inactive form rather than in the free, unbound form that interacts with estrogen receptors in breast tissue. Soy products, which include tofu, miso, tempe, soy milk, soy proteins, edamame (soybeans in the pod), have also been found to:

• Inhibit the formation of new blood vessels (angiogenesis) that can feed tumors.

• Have antioxidant activity that protect us from free radicals (see below).

- Limit the polyamines (forms of protein broken down in the body) required for cancer growth.

- Increase a self-programmed form of cell death known as apoptosis.

- Reduce insulin resistance, thereby decreasing levels of bio-available estrogen.

Research published in *AntiCancer Research* (May/June 1999) concluded that the use of genistein (one of the isoflavones found in soy) along with tamoxifen resulted in better cancer cell inhibition than tamoxifen alone. Because phytoestrogens behave like SERMs with fewer possible side effects, it appears that they may be the wave of the future in breast cancer risk reduction.

Soy is one of at least three hundred plants to have compounds with estrogenic activity. Many legumes, grains, nuts, and seeds are rich in sources of phytochemicals that act as estrogen adaptogens, meaning that they can act as antiestrogens or as estrogen agonists (behaving similarly to estrogen). Plant estrogens work by mimicking the activities of estrogen in our own bodies or by affecting estrogen metabolism. They can reduce the overstimulation of receptor sites by estrogen (acting as estrogen antagonists) or bind to receptors to exert a very weak effect compared to the body's own estrogens (acting as estrogen agonists).

Most of the research on soy has identified two isoflavone compounds known as *genistein* and *daidzein* as the phytochemicals most responsible for soy's anti-cancer activities. While most of us are familiar with isoflavones and look for them when we select soy products, most consumers still don't know that these two important compounds, genistein and daidzein, must be converted by healthy intestinal bacteria to active substances like equol, a phytoestrogen produced in the body. If your intestinal flora has been compromised by the use of antibiotics or drugs that increase intestinal pH, stress, diarrhea, intestinal infections, high-sugar and low-fiber diets, or intestinal toxins, you may be less capable of biotransforming your soy than others. Stool analysis can assess the health of your intestinal flora. Although a compromised intestinal flora may be asymptomatic, bloating, indigestion, changes in stool, such as diarrhea or constipation, body aches, fogginess, and poor concentration may indicate a need for an assessment. Ask your doctor to recommend a laboratory for testing.

Soy's anti-cancer properties don't stop at the popular isoflavones. Soy is replete with protease inhibitors, phytates, phytosterols, omega-3 and fatty acids, and phenolic acids, which have anti-cancer properties. The Bowman-Birk Inhibitor (BBI), a compound in soy foods that can block the action of specific enzymes that promote tumor growth, has proven soy's ability to prevent and inhibit the formation of cancer cells. Indeed, a more concentrated and potent form of BBI, called *BBIC*, has been given a designation of investigational New Drug Status and has undergone human trials.

How Much Soy Should You Eat?

Current recommendations call for eating at least 25 grams and not more than 60 grams of soy food daily. It appears that the benefits of soy accrue in this range. I recommend soy food and *not* supplemental isoflavones alone. Many of the conflicting research about soy results derive from the use of these isoflavones by themselves without the other balancing and synergistic constituents of whole soy food. Discuss the amount of daily soy food that is right for you with your health care professional.

Soy after Menopause and with Breast Cancer: The Controversy

The use of soy is not without controversy. It's clear that premenopausal women enjoy a net reduction in the strength of circulating estrogens because soy products contain a weaker estrogenlike compound. But what if you are a menopausal woman with other factors that put you at high risk for breast cancer? Since you no longer produce much estrogen, eating a high phytoestrogen diet could boost your total estrogen levels. If your breast is prepared for less estrogen at this time of life, but receives more estrogen due to supplemental or dietary increase of the plant compounds, might you not be subjecting your epithelial cells to unwanted stimulation?

It's true that a large body of long-term studies investigating this problem does not yet exist. I advise you to discuss the matter with your physician. However, based on my own clinical experience and a review of available research, we believe that the benefits of soy for the anti-estrogenic effects and their relief of menopausal symptoms, such as hot flashes, vaginal dryness, cholesterol moderation, and possible maintenance and increasing of bone density, outweigh speculative potential risk. Additionally, the lifelong work of respected scientists like Dr. Herman Adlecreutz, a physician of Finland's University of Helsinki, emphasizes that there simply is no evidence that the amount of phytoestrogens found in whole soy foods stimulates already-existing cancer or initiates cancer growth.

Lignans Can Help Reduce Your Risk

Like soy, flaxseeds contain compounds that contain both estrogenic and antiestrogenic activities. They are replete with a particular plant substance called a *lignan*, which is converted by intestinal flora into active forms with estrogenic effects. Once again, healthy bacteria in the gut are vital for overall health. Yet, the colonization of these bacterial strains can be sabotaged easily by certain medications. I advise you to consult with a professional knowledgeable about intestinal flora to determine if you might be a candidate for what has come to be known as *probiotic* (as opposed to antibiotic) supplementation. Stool analysis can help you determine if you are a candidate for probiotic supplementation.

Studies suggest that lignan compounds compete with stronger forms of estrogens for receptor sites and that they may help reduce excessive levels of circulating estrogens by stimulating production of sex hormone–binding globulin (SHBG) in the liver, which means that more estrogen might be circulating in the bound, inactive form rather than the free, active form.

Lignans can be found especially in flaxseeds, but they can also be found in whole grains, fruits, berries, and some seeds. If you use flaxseed meal or oil, use brands carried in opaque bottles that are refrigerated and dated for freshness. It's important to discuss dosage with your health care professional, but a generally recommended range of servings might be one or two tablespoons of flax oil per day. You can add it to food but never cook with this very fragile oil. If you choose flaxseed meal, use two to three teaspoons of flaxseed meal two to three times per day. However, if this product is new to your diet, begin with a much smaller dose and gradually increase at your own pace.

A Healthy Liver Contributes to Breast Health

I juice fruits and vegetables. I still eat meat, but much less, and I eat produce only if it's organic. Nutrition is important, especially if you have cancer. • Joan

Estrogens, like other steroid hormones, are transported from the bloodstream through the liver and into the bowel for disposal. To prevent recycling estrogen back into the body, there must be a healthy liver to help make estrogen water soluble for bowel elimination, and there must be adequate fiber in the bowels to bind with estrogen and escort it out of the body.

To reduce the toxic load on your liver, you can:

• Decrease or stop eating animal products, including meat and chicken. Growth hormones are injected into meat and chicken. These animals also feed on water and grain, which can be made impure by runoff from chemical fertilizers and pesticides, containing xenoestrogens that can mimic estrogen. If you must eat animal products, eat a limited amount of free-range, organic, and hormone-free products.

• Decrease or stop eating vegetable produce laced with hormones and pesticides. Most supermarkets carry organic produce, although it's important to try to buy foods that are not shipped long distances and altered to sustain travel.

• Decrease or stop drinking alcoholic beverages and unclean water, such as any source of water that may contain excess amounts of chemicals like chlorine or heavy metals. This may include tap water or even bottled or filtered water.

• Decrease or stop excess drugs, such as recreational drugs, the overuse of aspirin, and so forth.

• Drink plenty of clean water to improve detoxification. To find out if your local water is unclean, take a water sample from your tap into you water district or to an independent chemical testing lab. If your water is unclean, have a water filter system installed. Reverse osmosis is the best form of protection, but can be costly. Different types of filtration systems are used to filter different kinds of matter, so it's important to choose a system based on the analysis of your local water. The type of system you use will depend on the type of water you have.

• Consume appropriate amounts of fiber such as vegetables, fruit, and whole grains. Some people are sensitive to certain sources of fiber, such as foods in the grass family or glutens. If this is true for you, you may want to avoid wheat or oatmeal in favor of other types of grains. Likewise, if you have a diverticular condition, avoid seeds and nuts. Nuts and seeds should be eaten raw. Make sure that the products you buy are fresh and have not been sitting on the shelf for months in a plastic bag.

• Consume a proper amount of high-quality protein, including free-range omega-3 eggs and soy (if your physician approves). You can also buy specially engineered whey proteins that are ion-exchanged, micronized, and filtered. Check the label for product information. Some soy products are genetically engineered. At the time of this writing, the jury is still out on the question of whether it's harmful to consume genetically modified organisms (GMOs). Although there are no long-term studies yet, it stands to reason that it might be better to eat products that are free of GMOs, especially if you have cancer or are at high risk.

• Speak to your health care professional about your personal need for lipotropic agents, like choline, methionine, and cysteine, and about your need for vitamins and minerals. Physicians with a background in nutrition will be most helpful. Acupuncturists, naturopaths, and chiropractors may also be versed in nutrition.

Environmental Toxins and Your Breast Health

There are many chemicals in the environment that can mimic the actions of estrogen in our bodies and bind to estrogen receptor sites. Though banned in 1974, DDT, for example, remains in some sections of soil around this country. Medical research has confirmed that breast fat cells can absorb residues of DDT from the bloodstream and store it at concentrations seven hundred times greater than is found in the blood. And just as it is absorbed at high concentrations in human fat cells, it is concentrated in animal fat cells as well, which means it will accumulate in dietary animal fat. Consequently, it is advisable to buy pesticide-free and hormone-free meat and dairy products when possible, to buy organic products, to trim sources of animal fat before cooking, and to buy low-fat dairy products.

DDT is only one of many sources of xenoestrogens, or chemical estrogens, plaguing our modern world. Dioxin, a by-product of the industrial manufacture of chlorine and chlorine-based chemicals found in PVC plastics, chlorine-bleached paper, and other products is an undisputed oncogenic (cancer-causing) substance. Many similar toxic compounds poison the plastics, fuels, and pesticides we use. Check with research centers like the Center for Bioenvironmental Research at Tulane and Xavier universities for guidance. The website, www.cbr. tulane.edu, provides information about environmental toxins and their impact upon both the environment and human health. The center also developed a holistic research program to aid in disease prevention in humans and ecosystems. (This is an educational and not a prescriptive website.) These substances tend to be more aggressive than our own estrogenic compounds, and they tend to have a longer half-life in our bodies. Thus, they hang around to stimulate our tissues more tenaciously than even our own hormones, and our bodies have to work harder to detoxify and eliminate them.

Fats, Free Radicals, and Other Food Matters

• I recommend that you get most of your fat in the form of mono-unsaturated fats, like extra virgin olive oil and essential fatty acids in the omega-3 category found in cold-water fatty fish like salmon, tuna, mackerel, cod, sardines, and herring (not pickled), seeds, like flaxseed, and sea vegetables. Recently a report published in the *Archives of Internal Medicine* (vol. 158, no. 1, 1998) concluded that monounsaturated fat in the diet of more than 61,000 Swedish women ages 40 to 70 appeared to reduce the risk of breast cancer by 45 percent. Also, another study published in *Nutrition Research* (vol. 9, 1989) found that by increasing fish oils and flaxseed oil in the diets of mice lowered the incidence of breast cancer produced by exposure to a known carcinogen by more than 70 percent. Some researchers believe that while adding these oils is healthy, it is removing transfatty acids and the saturated animal fats from the diet that is most important. Others explain that the use of these fats blunts the estrogen response of cell receptors. It appears as though omega-6 fatty acids found in the highest proportion in vegetable oils, seed and nut oils (like sunflower and safflower seeds along with peanut, soybean, and sesame oils), margarine, most pastries, and breads amplify the estrogen signal in sensitive cells. Instead, use flax oil on foods (it is too fragile to use during any cooking) and cook with olive oil.

• Free radicals are reactive oxygen molecules that can destroy cells around the body and initiate the development of cancer. A free radical is a molecule that is unstable because it has an unpaired electron. To stabilize itself, this molecule frantically searches for another electron to complete the set, and it will steal an electron wherever it can. This electron piracy can mean damaging cellular structures. The membrane that surrounds the cell is often attacked first. But other parts of cells, including DNA, are vulnerable to attack. When DNA is damaged, cells can mutate and proliferate out of control, and thus become cancerous. Free radicals can come from the environment generated by cigarette smoke, automobile pollution, ultraviolet rays, and chemical pollutants. They can also be produced inside our bodies by the normal production of energy and white blood cells that attack pathogenic invaders, which can occur during an illness or any time your body encounters a substance that it recognizes as foreign. One way to diminish potential damage to our DNA from free radicals is to avoid chemical pollutants and other environmental toxins. Another is to provide our bodies with dietary antioxidants, which protect us from free radicals by lending one of their own electrons to the rampaging radicals. Examples of antioxidants found in food include the carotenes from dark-colored, green, orange, and yellow vegetables and fruits; lignans found in flaxseeds; whole grains; nuts and seeds; and flavonoids found in dark purple and red fruits and vegetables. Generally, I recommend eating five or more servings of fruits and vegetables of all colors each day. The closer you get to eating a rainbow of various vegetables and fruits, the more you will benefit from the plethora of plant chemicals they contain. These phytonutrients do more than quench free radicals. They increase cell-killing (cytotoxic) activity of cancer-detecting natural killer cells; inhibit the formation of neoplastic (tumor) cells through the presence of a substance called *glucarate* that regulates proper cell growth and inhibits the initiation of cancer; and stimulate enzymes that diminish the effect of estrogen. Important antioxidants include vitamins A, C, and E; coenzyme nutrients, like Coenzyme Q10; and other nutrient substances, like lipoic acid, glutathione, n-acetyl cysteine, and minerals, like selenium and other nutrients. Adding more cruciferous vegetables to your diet may increase cancer protection. These vegetables, which include broccoli, cabbage, bok choy, kale, kohlrabi, brussel sprouts, mustard greens, cauliflower, radishes, and others, contain indole-3-carbinol and sulforaphanes, which appear to have anticarcinogenic effects. Specifically, these reduce the amount of a particular kind of breakdown product of estrogen, 16-alpha-hydroxyestrone, which has been reported to be carcinogenic (see above). Heat may destroy some of the vital phytonutrients, so cook and steam these vegetables lightly.

• Garlic is rich in sulfur-containing amino acids, which are very important in detoxification, and they provide healthy doses of the protective mineral selenium. Garlic is also a standout among spices possibly due to its ability to stimulate an enzyme known to inhibit cancer initiation and growth known as *glutathione-S-transferase*. Consider adding garlic to your meals for flavor and protection.

• Drink green tea with those cancer prevention meals. It contains polyphenols and other antioxidants that reduce cellular membrane damage from free radicals, reduce DNA damage, increase serum sex hormone–binding globulin, and decrease serum estradiol levels. Estradiol is the most active form of estrogen.

• Do not use too much sugar. The overconsumption of sugar and refined carbohydrates increases the risk of several cancers, including breast and endometrial cancers. Not only do sugars rob our bodies of essential nutrients we need to maintain breast health and general wellness, they also stimulate the production of excess insulin. Insulin, the same hormone that enables us to bring glucose into our cells as a fuel source, also prompts the body to store fat. Higher insulin levels appear to correlate with increased fat storage, and increased fat storage creates fertile soil for increased estrogen production. Insulin and estrogen work synergistically to promote cell division. This increases the risk of cancers in certain people. Your body can influence insulin levels. Researchers believe that those of us with apple-shaped bodies, where excess fat is carried above the hips, are more at risk for higher insulin levels than those with pear-shaped bodies, where excess weight is carried on the thighs and buttocks. In order to reduce insulin to appropriate levels, I recommend that you exercise regularly, select omega-3–rich polyunsaturated fats and monounsaturated fats in place of saturated animal fats, eat the right amount of protein, consume at least 25 grams of fiber daily, and reduce pastries, excess sodium, breads, simple carbohydrates, processed foods, and processed grains.

A complementary approach to breast health takes a great deal about you into consideration. Your wellness depends upon choices you make about your emotions, social network, exercise, food, environment, and your body's ability to cleanse itself. In order to determine the right amount of fiber, protein, essential fatty acids, soy isoflavones, antioxidant foods, and nutrients for you individually, seek out a health care professional who is knowledgeable about nutrition, especially as it relates to women's health. Health care professionals as well as friends and colleagues may be able to provide referrals. I recommend a team approach to breast health, as prudent choices require a broad view of the problem. Do not forget, as well, that you might want to include on your health care team those professionals who can help you manage your life, its stresses, and your emotions. Henry David Thoreau wrote, "Nature is doing her best each moment to make us well. She exists for no other end. With the least inclination to be well, we should not be sick."

CHAPTER SEVENTEEN

Your Emotions after Breast Cancer: Detecting Depression

By Michelle B. Riba, M.D., M.S.

J. B. is a 53-year-old divorced woman with two teenage daughters. While there was no breast cancer in her family, on routine mammography, J. B. was found to have suspicious calcifications, which required further investigation. After some delay in seeing the surgeon due to the surgeon's vacation schedule, J. B. was found, on core biopsy, to have a two-centimeter invasive ductal carcinoma. She was given the option of sentinel lymph node mapping and a lumpectomy versus mastectomy. J. B. had 6/20 positive lymph nodes. Her tumor was ER positive, PR positive, and her2/neu negative. Treatment following surgery consisted of chemotherapy with Adriamycin and cytoxan, radiotherapy, and then five years of tamoxifen.

While J. B.'s coworkers and supervisors were sympathetic to her medical issues, the deadlines at work continued to either pile up or were given to others to do. J. B.'s teenagers were sometimes supportive and sometimes angry that J. B. was so tired and didn't have patience. They found their mother to be depressed and irritable. She no longer felt like cooking or shopping with them. They were embarrassed by how she looked after losing her hair. The girls often stayed at friends' houses and distanced themselves from J. B.

Prior to the breast cancer diagnosis, J. B. had started a new but promising relationship with C. M., but this was put on indefinite hold. J. B. didn't have the energy or desire to work on the relationship and didn't feel sexually attractive. At the same time, C. M. didn't seem invested in trying to help J. B. with her medical problems.

J. B. felt embarrassed by how she looked. She felt her breast was deformed; she tried various wigs and scarves but felt unattractive. The radiotherapy made her feel tired. She had gained about ten pounds after the chemotherapy and was having difficulty taking the weight off because she didn't have the energy for physical exercise. She felt fearful that she would be alone.

J. B. attended a support group in her town but the meeting frightened her. Several of the women in the group had metastatic disease or recurrent breast cancer. Thinking of a recurrence or a poor outcome was not helpful to J. B. at this time and she decided not to go back for a second session.

All of her physicians thought she was doing well, and from a medical point of view, she was doing well. But J. B. felt hopeless about the future and depressed about her vulnerability and the fate of her daughters should she have a recurrence. She didn't feel or look like her former self and was angry that this had happened to her. She was also fearful of any genetic predisposition to breast cancer that she might pass on to her daughters. It felt like people at work, her doctors, and her daughters just wanted her to "get over it" and move on with her life, but somehow she couldn't do that. J. B. felt depressed and worried. She couldn't sleep at night. She was eating more than she should and not exercising. J. B.. felt irritable and cried at least once a day. Mornings were difficult, and she found herself not wanting to get out of bed. Her friends stopped calling to ask her out for social activities.

•••

The emotional turmoil faced by J. B. is all too familiar. Many women with breast cancer say that dealing with the emotional aspects of cancer is as difficult, if not sometimes more difficult, than dealing with the physical changes. Within moments of hearing the results of her mammogram, J. B.'s life was forever changed. You may be feeling the same way.

Like J. B., your life may have been going well before you received your diagnosis. You may have felt, like she did, that you were in a trance as you listened to the unfamiliar medical terminology your doctors used when talking to you about your illness. You may be overwhelmed by the often incomprehensible technical information on breast cancer supplied by well-meaning friends and relatives, and you may be frightened by reading about all the possible outcomes of breast cancer.

Suddenly, it may seem as though you are no longer in control of your own life, but that you are being controlled by your doctors' schedules. Like J. B., you may have a difficult time asking questions about your treatment or seeking a second or third opinion. Although some of J. B.'s friends urged her to get more opinions about her treatment, J. B. felt this might damage her relationship with her doctors, and she didn't know if her HMO would pay for further opinions. Frankly, she didn't have the energy to seek other suggestions.

Likewise, she realized that she could no longer provide her daughters with the same interest and supervision that she did prior to breast cancer and was relieved that they began spending time with friends. Although she had started a new relationship, she no longer felt feminine and appealing.

Although her doctors pronounced her well after treatment, J. B. had become depressed. She had what we call *major depression* with:

- Decrease in energy

- Problems sleeping

- Weight gain

- Feeling hopeless and helpless

- Feeling tearful and experiencing mood changes

- Loss of pleasure in formerly enjoyable activities

- Trouble concentrating

- Suicidal thoughts

Although J. B. was not suicidal, she did wonder if her daughters would be better off without her. She didn't want to go out with friends and didn't enjoy things that she used to, such as going to the movies or biking. She was having trouble concentrating at work, and she felt irritable. She tried a support group, but it didn't help. She felt alone and worried.

The day after I was released from the hospital, I packed my suitcase and drove to a hotel. I couldn't stop crying. I hurt all over, and I was so tired. My husband found me and encouraged me to come home. I needed help. The next day I found a therapist and continued to cry for another week. Finally, I was put on an antidepressant drug and I started to feel better. • Dianne

Breast Cancer Can Change the Way You Feel about Yourself

Our self-image is often based on the way we look, how well we parent, and how well we perform at work. When it's no longer possible to maintain the same appearance or body image, when you can't work regular hours or can't go to your children's functions, your sense of self may suffer a blow. You may not feel like the same person you used to be, and others may perceive you differently. It may be hard to know when, if ever, you will feel the same again.

Although your body may look and feel different, the impact of breast cancer and chemotherapy are often hidden from view. Walking around in public with a wig, hat, or scarf may feel like you are holding up a red flag to signal your experience. One of the worst things about going out, for many women, is seeing the worried or pitiful looks on others' faces, and many women stop going to church or synagogue for this reason.

Women cope with changes in their appearance in different ways, including wearing wigs around their significant others. One of the women I treated told me that her husband loved her new wig. She was a bit upset by this because, of course, the wig was artificial. Some women wear teddies or cover-ups after breast surgery. A partner's approval of these additions to the wardrobe can be confusing. Another woman I saw in my practice chose to buy very glittery, dazzling garments, clothes that she would never have worn before. She decided that if people were going to stare at her anyway, she would really give them something to stare at! She had fun shopping, and her sisters enjoyed getting new hats, vests, and jewelry to coordinate with her new outfits.

The clothes or wigs we use to hide or dramatize changes in our appearance often have more to do with helping others to cope with cancer than with making ourselves feel better, as it's frequently women's plight to worry or care about others, even when faced with situations that make us vulnerable. Rather than worrying about what other people feel, we must learn to take time to think about how we can best care for ourselves. If you begin to feel better about yourself, your children and significant other will pick up on that and feel better, too. It's hard to switch gears suddenly and focus on yourself and your body, but if ever there was a time to do it, now is that time.

You and Your Family

Many women with breast cancer feel tremendous guilt. While it may not be rational or logical, some women feel responsible for disrupting the family's normal routine, and women who are mothers are especially vulnerable to this feeling. Not being able to be "supermom" all the time can be difficult, and some turn their feelings inward. Sometimes mothers allow their children's responses to their illness to complicate their own guilt and anger at the disease. Many mothers already feel guilty, for example, if they also work outside the home, use baby-sitters, or are not around as much as they would like to be. If you are feeling guilty, it can be useful to try to sort out where those feelings are coming from and whether or not they are really rational. Feelings of mild guilt are generally "normal," but these feelings can be unhealthy when taken to extremes.

Some women avoid going to their children's plays or sports activities because they don't want to embarrass them by the way they look. One of my patients didn't go to her child's confirmation rehearsal because her wig wasn't ready yet, and her daughter didn't want her mother to be seen with a scarf. Going to the rehearsal would have been a way to teach her child and her friends that we can't look perfect all the time. Walking into the rehearsal room to let the kids know that she was okay and still

TALKING TO YOUR CHILDREN ABOUT ILLNESS

For many parents, talking to a child about serious illness is a difficult task. We're not always sure how to begin or what to say. If you need help, consider that:

- Teachers and school counselors can often guide parents in learning how to talk to their children.

- Some schools have medical support groups for children whose parents have significant medical problems.

- Some cancer centers have age-appropriate groups for children of parents with cancer.

- Libraries and organizations like the American Cancer Society are good resources as well.

the same great mom as she always had been would have been a useful coping response. Bringing cookies or brownies to the rehearsal might have helped to break the ice.

Children can become depressed or anxious themselves when someone in the family is ill. Younger children, especially, may start to act out in school or have difficulty at night. Separation from the mother due to medical treatment is particularly hard. Even young children know that there is something new or different going on in the household. What and how much you should tell your child has to do with your child's developmental stage, chronological age, and the questions your child asks. It's harmful for children to hear their parents and other family members whispering and "telling secrets," or to hear information from other children. When this happens, a child feels betrayed not to have been included in family discussions from the start.

> We realized that we could create a lot of fear by withholding information, so my husband and I felt it was important to share with our children that I had cancer. It was difficult to know just how much to share. My oldest instantly responded with sobs, but we were able to reassure her that there were a lot of good treatments, that I was going to be okay, and that it was just going to take a while. • Linda L.

Spouses and significant others most often rally to the aid of the woman with breast cancer, or they can become emotionally troubled. You and your significant other may experiences changes in sexual activity. Your hormonal status may change, and chemotherapy may have a negative effect on your sexual feelings and interest in sex. Similarly, depression and anxiety can greatly affect your libido and desire for sex, as do many of the antidepressants currently in use. Other issues facing loved ones include, but are not limited to, increased chores and burdens at home, financial issues, and anticipatory grief and loss.

It is often helpful to have your spouse or significant other attend some medical appointments with you and to schedule some time alone with your doctor or nurse practitioner to ask questions. As a psychiatrist, I try to have at least one meeting with each couple and to ask specifically about sex, libido, and other issues around sexuality. I find that most of my patients don't place the same value on sex during treatment as they did before, but they do worry about whether their partner's needs are being fulfilled.

My husband. What an incredible man! I really felt I was able to get through all of my surgeries and treatments so well because of the constant loving encouragement he gave me. He reassured me that he loved me and not my body. The experience of having cancer has brought us all closer. When you realize how temporary life is, you start to value what is most important. The most important thing we have on earth is our relationships. • Linda L.

When I was first diagnosed, my husband got on the Internet and read an article about men who were dealing with a significant other diagnosed with breast cancer. The article explained that the first thing many men want to do is to turn inward. It helped him to realize that this wasn't going to be the best response. • Francine

My daughter has been braver and stronger than any child should have to be. She was three when I first got cancer. She doesn't remember a time before Mommy was sick. Sometimes I think that's really sad, but more often I hope that she takes cancer and uses it to learn about strength and commitment. My husband has been really wonderful, too. There was never a doctor's visit or an anxious moment when he wasn't there. There was never a time when he didn't feel and act as though I was the most attractive woman in the world. • Joelle

Your Stage of Life May Affect the Way You Respond to Your Diagnosis

Lucy is a 30-year-old woman who is a bank vice president in the Midwest. She and her husband were married for two years and were thinking about starting a family when Lucy felt a lump in her right breast during her morning shower. Coming from a large family, Lucy couldn't imagine being childless. With every doctor's appointment, she raised this issue as her primary concern. The physicians tried to get her to concentrate on the cancer and its treatment, but her worry about the impact of chemotherapy and radiotherapy on her chances of having children were of utmost importance to her.

•••

Certainly, your stage of life has a good deal to do with your emotional response to breast cancer. In general, we tend to think of younger women as having a more serious course of illness and facing stage-of-life issues with more difficulty. If you are in your twenties or thirties, you may be thinking about getting into a new relationship and having children, and you may have to face different issues than an older woman. I've worked with women who were diagnosed with breast cancer when they were planning their weddings, and we were able to work the chemotherapy and possible hair loss around the date of the wedding and honeymoon. Similarly, women who are pregnant at the time of diagnosis must determine with their doctors how to time their surgery and other treatments around the pregnancy.

Women with breast cancer who want children may have to face very difficult discussions of banking eggs, in vitro fertilization, surrogate carriers, and adoption. Decision-making is often very hard when such emotionally charged issues arise. It's not uncommon for women to worry about their ability to conceive after breast cancer and to worry about whether or not they might be suitable adoptive parents, given the cancer diagnosis. Women also worry about finding a new partner after cancer and whether their new partner will accept them and their appearance as well as the possibility of a recurrence.

Older women often have additional burdens, such as caring for a spouse or partner who also has medical problems. Some of the older women I have seen in my practice opted for mastectomy rather than breast-saving surgery and radiation because they didn't have time to be away from their infirm husbands. If you are an older woman with cancer, you may worry about how your husband or partner will fare without you. One woman I saw as a patient bought her husband a nice suit and tie to wear at her funeral. She was worried he wouldn't look nice, and she didn't want to be embarrassed! Three years later when she was still around, I asked her husband if the suit still fit. Thinking that you won't be able to see your grandchildren grow, graduate from school, and get married can also be very disheartening and sad.

Dealing with the Loss of a Breast(s) or Changes in Appearance

Women have different feelings and attachments to their breasts. Some women and their partners use their breasts in lovemaking more than others. Some women breast-fed their children and were perhaps breast-fed themselves. Some women really enjoy their figures, and the way their breasts look. Others have always felt themselves flat-chested or have had sagging, large breasts that were very noticeable. In other words, the breast means different things to all of us.

No matter what you feel about your breast, losing a breast or breasts to cancer or having surgery done, as with lumpectomy, is a major trauma. Some women cope better with breast cancer surgery and its consequences if they have plastic reconstructive surgery done immediately or soon after initial surgery. Others don't want to face any more surgery than they have to. Still others are fearful of any operation and of having general anesthesia. Many women worry about having lymphedema and never looking quite right in bathing suits and certain types of dresses.

It's important to talk about these fears and worries with your doctor and to weigh these issues alongside considerations that will offer you the most positive health outcome in the long run. You may also benefit from talking to other breast cancer survivors or to a therapist or psychiatrist who has helped women with this issue. Every woman feels differently about the loss of her breast(s) or a change in their appearance. Your feelings may arise from thoughts about how you will look with or without clothing, the way a change in appearance may affect your sense of well-being in relationships and in lovemaking, and how you feel about surgery. Tell those around you how you feel and what you need to help you through this life-altering experience.

Why Is It So Hard to Recognize Emotional Problems Linked to a Breast Cancer Diagnosis?

As we've seen, emotional challenges related to breast cancer are common and not at all surprising. What is surprising is that women are not regularly asked about their emotional life and how they are coping with cancer. The reasons why are complex. There's a lot going on medically and surgically, especially at the beginning of treatment. Surgical procedures and medical tests must be scheduled; arrangements must be made at home for the care of other family members; and your work schedule and deadlines may have to be reevaluated, if you work outside the home.

The truth is that many women know they are depressed, but don't tell their doctors because they're worried that the doctors' knowledge of their anxiety and depression might affect their treatment. For example, some women worry that less chemotherapy might be prescribed because of their vulnerability.

There is also a stigma attached to mental illness, even if it arises in connection with a cancer diagnosis. Some people worry that they already have one serious problem to contend with and that by admitting to

---

UNTREATED DEPRESSION IS SERIOUS

Untreated depression and anxiety can be quite serious over time and should be treated by a physician. Depression and anxiety affects your quality of life and the lives of those around you. It affects adherence to medication and other treatments, such as seeing your doctor regularly, and even checking on other health concerns, such as getting yearly pap smears.

When depressive symptoms, such as problems with concentration, suicidal thoughts, decreased energy, changes in appetite, sleep, mood, decreased interest in formerly enjoyable activities, guilt feelings, agitation, or slowed movements last more than two weeks, consult with your physician or mental health professional. Depression is highly treatable. Do not delay in addressing this important health concern.

depression that, they may have to take an antidepressant or anxiolytic, which may or may not be true. Some are concerned about environmental or other causes of cancer and fear that the medication may be impure or contribute to a possible recurrence. Because many people don't want to take these medications, they turn to complementary or alternative medications without telling their doctors, imagining that their doctors will object or be angry. It's very helpful to ask your doctor, up front, about his or her attitude toward complementary regimens. Most doctors these days ask about alternative treatments and want to have a dialogue about this with their patients.

Let your doctor know if you have had a problem with depression, anxiety, or substance abuse in the past—you're not alone. There's about a 30 percent chance of having one of these problems during your lifetime.[1] If you're like many, you may feel embarrassed about disclosing this information to your doctor. You may worry that it will be included on your medical records or that others, including insurers, will see it. This is a reasonable concern, one that you should discuss with your doctor at the very beginning of treatment.

Who Should Watch for Emotional Problems?

Because there are so many caregivers involved in treating breast cancer, it's sometimes unclear who should be in charge of thinking about the emotional health of patients. Many times, if you don't "fall apart" in the doctor's office, no one knows you are having a difficult time. There is a range of means to address emotional difficulties from educational resources to treatment with a mental health professional or another counselor, such as a pastoral counselor. Depending on the type of distress you are experiencing and clinical diagnosis, psychotherapy and/or medication may be recommended.

---

[1] Kessler, R.C., McGonagle, K.A., Swartz, M., Blazer, D.G., Nelson, C.G., "Sex and depression in the National Comorbidity Survey I: Lifetime prevalence, chronicity and recurrence." *Journal of Affective Disorders* 1993 (19) 85–96.

What Should You Do if You Are Experiencing Distress?

The gold standard for treating the emotional aspects of cancer requires that each patient and situation be approached as unique with an individualized treatment plan. Nonetheless, there are certainly aspects of care that should be standard:

• There should be a routine, regular system for asking about emotions and distress. Clinicians can use standardized scales, symptom inventories, or questionnaires that you and your family can complete. Ideally, you should be assessed for emotional challenges at all visits. Your physicians should make you feel comfortable talking about anxiety, depression, sexuality, substance abuse, and issues regarding family members, and you should be referred to someone who can fully understand and help you and your family.

• Care by a good mental health practitioner should always be available to you. This can be a psychiatrist, social worker, or psychologist. Breast cancer centers and individual oncologists and surgeons

| CHOOSING A GOOD THERAPIST: TIPS

• Who does your oncologist recommend?

• Does the therapist have experience working with patients with cancer and their families? However, it is not always necessary to see someone who works with cancer patients.

• Is the therapist part of your managed care or behavioral mental health plan?

• Does the therapist have flexible hours?

• Choose a physician or therapist who can listen and who values the doctor-patient relationship.

• Think about choosing a therapist who is known for respecting and understanding cultural differences.

• Seeing a psychiatrist for initial evaluation is best. Further treatment can be arranged thereafter.

should be able to easily refer you to such professionals and should communicate with them about your emotional health.

Medication is not needed to treat all depression and anxiety. But most medications for depression and anxiety today are very safe and effective when used appropriately. Although a primary care physician can prescribe medications such as antidepressants (like fluoxetine, sertraline, and citalopram), anxiolytics (such as lorazepam, clonazepam, and alpraxolam), and sleep medications, many people need various forms of psychotherapy while they are battling breast cancer. Psychotherapeutic interventions between a therapist and a patient with cancer focus on trying to improve your morale, self-esteem, and coping strategies. Specific types of interventions include but are not limited to:

• **Brief supportive therapy.** In this type of therapy, the therapist takes an active, supportive stance to help you focus on your concerns about this illness.

• **Cognitive-behavioral therapy.** This type of therapy offers a realistic focus on stressors, problems, and ways of coping.

• **Psychodynamic insight-oriented therapy.** Here the goal is to help you understand how your past relationships might affect your current ability to cope with the cancer.

• **Behavioral therapies.** These therapies include progressive relaxation, guided imagery, meditation, biofeedback, and hypnosis.

• **Substance abuse counseling.** Many people have addictions and dependence on alcohol, tobacco, prescription drugs, and street drugs. Addictions can affect cancer treatment, if not addressed by appropriate professionals.

• **Marital and family therapy.** You and your family members may seek counseling to help resolve issues brought up by the illness and improve communication.

• **Pastoral counseling.** Talking to your clergyperson can also be helpful. Some clergy people are also licensed psychologists or social workers.

| CAN GROUP THERAPY HELP YOU?

Group therapy is an important part of good cancer care. Dr. David Spiegel pioneered supportive/expressive groups for breast cancer patients, showing that those who are in such groups have a better quality of life and may even live longer. Dr. Fawzy I. Fawzy did similar work with patients with melanoma. Rather than function as support groups where patients "drop in" primarily for education and support, supportive/expressive groups include patients of similar diagnosis, gender, or other identifiers who are chosen to be part of an organized therapeutic experience. The group becomes an opportunity to share feelings and emotions under the guidance and supervision of trained therapists.

But groups are not for everyone. Some women don't want to be in a group where everyone is talking about cancer. The severity of the patients in the group J. B. attended scared her. She might have done much better if her doctors helped her find a supportive/expressive group of patients in her stage of illness. The training of the therapist who is leading the group is important. Certainly, you want to choose someone with formal mental health training who is experienced in leading groups. It would be helpful if your doctor or other clinician, such as your nurse, could work with you to determine the best group and therapist for you. You can also call the American Cancer Society at 1-800-ACS-2345, or visit its website (http://www.cancer.org) for more information on choosing a support group or group therapy sessions in your area. (See the resource directory at the end of this book.)

• **Group therapy.** This type of therapy allows women to face issues with members of the group who have similar experiences. In group therapy, women with cancer have the opportunity to address their unknown future together.

Using the Internet for Information and Support

The Internet has been a boon to patients, allowing easy access to a wealth of information and chat rooms for advice and support. But timing is everything. There are times when information is useful and times when it's not. As with J. B., friends and relatives may provide information that is not appropriate to your particular medical problem, and it may become difficult to wade through all the technical aspects of treatment and to learn how to read scientific papers overnight. It may be hard, but you must let your loved ones know how much and how little information you want from the Internet. I recommend avoiding websites that are not sanctioned by known and trusted organizations.

Some of us intellectualize our feelings, often as a defense against anxiety and worry. While it's important to ask questions and be prepared for your medical visits, it's equally important to realize that you have a right to your individual feelings about cancer and need not be stoic or bury your feelings. Taking charge of your medical care is a vital tactic in dealing with cancer, but it can also be a coping mechanism with limits. You must care for your emotional self as much as for your physical body.

> You wouldn't believe the number of books and articles I received. You name it, I've got it. The amount of information you may be supplied with is overwhelming. It's important to ask your doctor about the information you receive, because you will hear so many differing opinions. You will have to ask some people to stop, and with others you will have to politely nod and say thank you. We don't yet know how to use the amount of information available to us, and it can often be very scary.
> • Francine

> One of the first things I did when I first felt the lump was to go on the Internet. I did hours and hours of research. My sister is a four-year survivor, so she helped me. I think it's important to do your own research, always get a second opinion, and talk to other women. • Anne

Letting Your Friends and Family Know What You Need

As we've discussed, women are used to taking care of other people—our parents, children, husbands, lovers, boyfriends, and girlfriends. Asking for help is unfamiliar. It's tough to ask others to bring in food for the family, to drive the carpool, or to ask husbands and friends to clean the house. You may have to ask for rides to chemotherapy or radiation treatments, or take time off work. Doing so without feeling guilt is a

IF SOMEONE YOU CARE ABOUT HAS BREAST CANCER

- Don't wait until your friend or relative asks you for something, tell her what you will do. For instance, you can say, "I am going to pick up your groceries this week. I'll get the list from your husband," or "I'm going to bring your children to and from Sunday school for the next three months."

- Many women with breast cancer feel isolated when friends stop calling, thinking that they don't want to bother them. Sending cute cards or thoughtful notes can be helpful.

- Bringing food or treats for the family is often appreciated.

- Ask what you can do to help, and keep asking. Needs change over time.

tremendous challenge. If you identify as a "superwoman," one who is always capable of responding to and filling others' needs, understand that asking for help is okay. It's a sign of resourcefulness and strength, not dependence and weakness.

I have had amazing support, but relationships can be challenging after a cancer diagnosis. My oldest son had some difficulty with my diagnosis and was afraid to see me for the longest time. It took a lot to figure out why, but he was afraid. Now he is totally different and very helpful. As a person newly diagnosed with cancer, you will get many different reactions, and you will have to understand what is happening with each person. At the same time, you have to be careful about what you take in and how you let it affect you. · Francine

I have four teenagers who helped quite a bit and were very supportive. They would do things around the house that needed to be done, especially during chemotherapy. My husband did the laundry or had the kids do it. If you need help, ask for it. If you ever considered having a cleaning crew in to do the house, now is the time to do it. · Anne

If someone you know has breast cancer, you can do many things for her. You can clean, bring the family a meal, take the kids for a day, give her a book on cancer, or just be there for her. You can just take two minutes to send a card in the mail. You don't know how much that means to someone, how much it can cheer that day up. · Linda L.

People May Let You Down

You may be disappointed by how some friends react to your illness. There are those who will stick with you through thick and thin and others who worry about "catching" the cancer or who have their own issues and can't be helpful. Recognizing that some friends are not going to be a part of your recovery can be a very difficult, disappointing, and significant part of your illness.

Where Can You Go for More Help?

There are excellent resources available to women with breast cancer. The Reach to Recovery Program offers guidance from other women who have had breast cancer. Many institutions have peer counselor programs, which allow you to get help and advice from another patient who is being treated for similar disease problems. Additionally, the American Cancer Society has an excellent peer-mentor program, where patients can speak to survivors who have been trained to answer questions and be helpful. You can ask your doctor, nurse, or social worker about getting help through these programs, which offer a wonderful and empathic way to ask questions and get answers from someone who has been through similar situations. The Look Good, Feel Better program gives women a chance to meet with professionals who can provide advice about cosmetics and hair. You can find out about all of these programs through your breast cancer center or hospital, or by calling the American Cancer Society listed in the resource directory.

What's Normal? What's Abnormal?

Many women wonder what is normal and what is abnormal when it comes to their emotional responses to breast cancer. They wonder what their significant others, children, and friends are feeling. It's understandable to want to return to the way things were before breast cancer, to be your "normal self" again. But now there is a "new normal." This new normal doesn't have to be better or worse than it was before your diagnosis. It's a matter of weighing your new experiences and the situations you've encountered and making adjustments.

You don't always have to be positive and upbeat to heal. It's true that we all do better when we are optimistic and participate in our health care, but it's not appropriate to feel this way all of the time. It is important to lay your worries and concerns on the table with a caring compassionate physician. Working within your doctor-patient relationship, you can discuss fears and concerns and, with guidance, reach this state of new normal.

Checkups following radiologic studies are always nerve-racking. In my practice, I talk with women before these visits, anticipating worries and concerns. Sometimes we schedule mental health visits before or after follow-up oncology or radiology appointments. I know some people will have problems sleeping before these visits, and I may do interventions, either with medication or telephone consultations. Sometimes small doses of antianxiety medication can be used to ease the stress and tension.

You have to realize that this is a very long journey you've started. You go through stages from "Why me?" to being very angry that it is you. If you can just accept that this is it, that you have been handed this in life, you can begin to take one day at a time. Don't think about the next ten to fifteen years. It's not going to be over in a month, but it is something that you have to do, just like anything, like going to the market. • Beverly

Nothing felt as it had before. I had to tell myself that very little was as it had been before and that it had saved my life. I want to emphasize that I was lucky to have lots of support. I don't know how I would have managed without the loving care and concern of my family, friends, and coworkers. • Teresa

My surgeon gave me the confidence that everything was going to be okay. He looked me dead in the eye and in a gentle way told me that I had cancer. My first thought was, "This is not going to beat me." Before I was diagnosed, I thought if I heard I had cancer, I wouldn't know what

I would do. Now I'm a Reach to Recovery volunteer, and I go out and I help people. Cancer was the start of a new life for me. · Linda R.

Life after Cancer

Returning to health or to a state of new normalcy after a diagnosis of cancer is one of the most difficult periods for patients. Although your physical appearance may be returning to "normal," facing and dealing with cancer is a life-altering experience that changes how you look at things. Priorities shift. Many of my patients have told me that work is no longer meaningful or that attaining tenure or a promotion doesn't seem quite as important. Likewise, getting back to a fulfilling sexual life isn't always the highest priority. Some women want to stay in their breast cancer support groups, while their spouses can't understand why they need to "hang on" to a cancer diagnosis. Children expect the same vim and vigor that their moms had before the cancer treatment. Often the fatigue of cancer takes months to dissipate after all the treatment is finished. But fatigue can also mask depression, so it's important to check in on how you're feeling.

Having cancer is frightening and lonely. Trying to get back into life as usual after cancer and its treatment can be every bit as frightening and lonely. It is important to remember that support and professional help are available. Tell your doctor, loved ones, and friends if you think that you are continuing to have emotional problems so that they can be professionally identified and treated, and you can begin to resume the life you want to lead.

CHAPTER EIGHTEEN

Becoming Strong at the Broken Places: A Guide to Suffering in Style

By Judith Harris, M.A., M.F.T.

The world breaks everyone and some become strong at the broken places. • Ernest Hemingway

All sorrows in life can be borne, if we tell a story about them.
• Karen Blixen

I work with clients who have stepped into the "wrong story." A life-threatening illness isn't what they thought they would experience. It isn't what they expected from life. Arnold Beiser, M.D., points out in his inspirational book *Flying Without Wings* that when life doesn't live up to our expectations, we always think there is something wrong with life, never with our expectations. However, the only thing we can control is our expectations, our thoughts, what we tell ourselves about what is happening. The more we can tell our stories, the more we can begin to see our deep connection to the universal concerns: growing up, handling relationships between parents and children, taking responsibility, developing a code of morality, and facing fear, abandonment, separation, and acceptance. The more we can listen to others' stories, the more we can realize that these fears, issues, and concerns are not ours alone. These issues are at the base of our fears when confronting illness and loss.

I was trained as a teacher and psychotherapist and have always been fascinated by how we become who we are, how we grow through pain. My professional experience—as a medical social worker, grief and trauma counselor, and mental health consultant to people dealing with various aspects of life-threatening illness—has shown me the resiliency of the human spirit and taught me the power of humor, as well as what it means to "suffer in style"—that is, to sustain a sense of optimism in the face of adversity. I am also a cancer survivor. My personal mission is to take the lessons learned from my clients' experiences and my own to help us improve both our capabilities and "copeabilities." In this chapter, I revisit some of those lessons to provide comfort, hope, perspective, and inspiration to those who have had a cancer diagnosis.

A cancer diagnosis triggers an identity crisis. We ask, "Who are we now?" How we take and survive the journey of cancer can help to define and redefine who we are for ourselves, our friends, and our family. As we move through this passage, we can become transformed from victim to victor and become the hero of our own adventure. Heroism has many forms and it doesn't mean being stoic or unaffected by cancer.

I've often heard clients say, "I'm not handling this well. I cry easily. I can't concentrate. I feel out of control." As if there were rules about handling a life-threatening illness without emotional disruption. Complaining, moaning, and whining are a part of life; just don't expect anything to change as a result of it. Lily Tomlin once said, "Man developed language from his innate need to complain." I congratulate my clients for understanding what a life-changing event they are facing and facing it with a range of emotions. As Elie Weisel stated, "A sane response to an insane situation is insane."

He that has a why to live for can bear any how. · Nietzsche

When things go wrong, we search for answers. I have never worked with a cancer survivor who did not seek to understand, "Why me?" if not, "Why now?" One of the main lessons I've learned is that human beings would rather feel guilty than helpless, so we search for reasons for our suffering. We would rather believe that there was something we did or didn't do that created our illness. Unfortunately, we often tell ourselves that we're being punished for some transgression and that we must be bad or we must be lacking something: "If I only had . . ." "I took hormones." "I was too stressed." "I ate too much of this and not enough of that." In fact, loss, change, illness, and accidents are part of a full life and are not devastating events from which we cannot recover. In a full life, joy and pain go hand in hand. It is important to know that we are always dealing with loss; someone or something is not the way we want it to be. The manner in which we receive sorrow will affect, good or bad, our subsequent life. In fact, the difference between a happy life and an unhappy life is the way each person comes to terms with loss.

The leading cause of stress is reality. • Jane Wagner

It's vital to mental health to see life as it is, not how we would like it to be. The common denominator in all emotional pain is feeling the need to change current reality. Unfortunately, we don't get to choose the challenges that life presents; we only get to choose how we are going to deal with them. The real challenge is not adding pain to life by the way we handle adversity. Cancer is a boundary experience: we feel "twice born," confronted with our existential situation. It is a complex disease we are only beginning to understand. It makes us feel different, isolated, and a stranger in our own lives. So much is the same, and yet everything has changed. When our bodies fail us, we no longer feel in control of our lives and realize the fact of our mortality. Maintaining emotional strength in the face of physical decline is not easy, but there are many resiliency skills that can be learned from other survivors.

Give sorrow words. The grief that does not speak whispers the o'er fraught heart and bids it break. • William Shakespeare

There is a complex relationship between the mind and body. They can become powerful allies in healing as demonstrated by the placebo effect, which has positive expectations as its only ingredient. Unfortunately, knowledge of the mind-body connection has created what Ken Wilber calls neotrogenic guilt, or New Age guilt, the concept that "I created my illness" by my thoughts. Now we worry when we have negative feelings or when we don't feel positive about our diagnosis or future. In reality, the mind-body connection is much more complicated than thought equals change or that thoughts cause physiological change. It is important for cancer survivors to know that research has shown that there is a difference between negative feelings and a negative mood. Negative moods are more pervasive and accompanied by negative thoughts about one's self, one's future, and one's ability to control things. The only negative feelings that affect the immune system are those we keep bottled up. There is therapeutic value in telling our story.

Experiencing genuine grief—sobbing and wailing—expresses the acceptance of our helplessness to do anything about our losses. As Proust reminds us, "We are healed of a suffering only by experiencing it in full." When we speak to other survivors, we become a part of the human comedy rather than the human tragedy and we learn that we have not been singled out for special punishment.

Expecting life to treat you fairly because you're a good person is like expecting a bull not to attack you because you're a vegetarian. • Rabbi Kushner

Cancer has the power to destroy our assumption that life is fair. Intellectually, we know life isn't fair, but when faced with a life-challenging diagnosis, our basic beliefs about the world are shattered, violated, and invalidated. That kind of life shock is a soul-shaking experience. Sometimes we cling to the belief that, "Limits, aging, death may apply to others but not to me." Unfortunately, if we don't accept that life isn't fair, we could spend time trying to figure out why we're being punished rather than spending time productively, and we could become bitter. Bitterness can lead to hopelessness and helplessness, which is so dangerous when confronting illness.

Everything can be taken from a man but the last of human freedoms to choose one's attitude in any given set of circumstances . . . one's own way. • Viktor Frankl, M.D.

There are certain beliefs, attitudes, and styles of thinking that can transform our pain into valuable lessons and diminish rather than add to our grief. Out of survivorship can come something worth salvaging—wisdom, strength. How am I the wiser? Stronger? Patience, perspective, courage, and faith lead us to mine the gifts of our grief. And our perspective on ourselves, our explanatory style, our theory about our past, our future, and our place in the world affects every area of our life. By reexamining our life, we can contact our core self, the "I" in the storm, which is our source of empathy, compassion, and strength. This is the timeless and ageless aspect of our true selves that reminds us that we are not our disease. We are bigger than anything that can happen to us. I am grateful and awed by my clients who have shown me that courage is not a single event but a daily struggle, and I have been privileged to see my clients sustain a sense of optimism in the face of great adversity.

In the midst of winter I discovered there was within me an invincible summer. • Albert Camus

Salvatore Maddi, Ph.D., and Suzanne Kasaba are psychologists who did stress research with healthy executives. They were among the first to study why people stay healthy rather than why they get sick. They identified what they called hardy personalities, people who thrive in the midst of stress. Hardiness is a set of beliefs people have about themselves, their world, and their place in it. Anyone can adopt these qualities of hardiness and effect change in their own life. The three Cs of hardiness are control, challenge, and commitment. It's very important to know where we believe our locus of control is—whether we believe we are controlled by outside forces or from within. Optimism and self-efficacy, our belief in our ability to handle our challenges, are crucial to good health. Pessimists view problems as pervasive, permanent, and personal, which causes them to give up in the face of challenge, allowing their beliefs to become self-fulfilling prophecies. Optimists are committed to something outside of themselves—family, faith, or a philosophy that gives their lives meaning. Optimism is a learned skill that allows us to look for solutions in the face of adversity.

Hardy personalities view change as a natural part of life. They don't try to fight what comes, and they let go of what goes. One of the most important tools for "suffering in style" is to resign as general manager of the universe. If we refuse to accept the world as it is, we miss out on any opportunities for happily-ever-after moments. I had a client who was very prominent in the film industry and had won awards. Yet he didn't feel good about himself because he thought he was too short. I told him to hold out and not be happy until he got taller. He was able to laugh with me about it because when it's stated that way, it sounds silly. What's not funny is that many of us hold on to things that can't be changed, and we use them as a source of unhappiness. I guarantee that if there is a conflict between the way the world is and the way we want it to be, if we persist with wanting to change those things that cannot be changed, we will never be happy.

We don't laugh because we're happy, we're happy because we laugh.
· William James

There's a Yiddish story that says after God created Adam, Adam was complaining about how vulnerable He had left him: "You gave the birds the gift of flight, you gave the lion strength, the horses speed, but you left me defenseless." God replied, "I gave you something more valuable than flight, strength, and speed. I gave you something that will also help you with yourself. I gave you a sense of humor." It has been said that man is the only animal that needs a sense of humor because man is the only animal that knows the difference between what is and what could have been. Humor is the soul's weapon against the unfairness of life. Frank Pittman, M.D., put it best when he said, "Laughter is the breath of life, the exclamation that you have discovered an alternative to death and despair . . ." It's not a way out but a way through it. Humor allows us to take back control and helps us to realize that we are bigger than our problems.

When the Heart weeps for what it has lost the Soul rejoices for what it has found. · Sufi proverb

There are undeniable benefits to having the myth of our immortality exploded. While death destroys the physical body, the concept of death can save us and give meaning to our lives. When we accept the inevitability of death, we realize we can't spend years waiting for life to begin at some future time when all our problems have been solved. Simultaneously, we can battle an illness and accept death as part of our lives. Accepting the world as it is and battling illness are not mutually exclusive. Battling illness is only possible once we accept that we have the illness.

Cancer can be an instant cure for neuroses. The reality of life suddenly becomes important. Many clients realign their priorities. I have seen clients finally able to say "no" without feeling guilty. Some feel liberated; finally they have permission to take care of themselves and do more of what they want to do.

When we are confronted by our mortality, we often find ourselves awakened to life's deepest questions. In fact, serious illness often motivates people to seek healing of the spirit. However, we learn that being healed is not the same as being cured. Healing is a process of becoming whole—physically and psychologically—which is in our control. Being cured is not something that everyone can achieve.

Spirituality, our deepest sense of connectedness and belonging to life, is an impulse toward unity, which is characterized by love, peace, creativity, and joy. True spirituality is the opposite of separation. When we are connected to life, we begin to see how our pain relates to the pain of others. Often with cancer, there is an enhanced sense of living in the immediate present, and we learn to let go of the guilty past and stop worrying about a fearful future. I'm reminded of a *Peanuts* cartoon, where Linus tells Charlie Brown, "I guess it's wrong always to be worrying about tomorrow. Maybe we should think only about today." Charlie replies, "No, that's giving up. I'm still hoping that yesterday will get better." Yesterday will never get better. The only thing we can change about the past is the way we look at it. In order to heal, it is imperative that we relinquish our wish to change the past. In fact, a good definition of forgiveness is giving up our need to have a happy past. Once we have let go of yesterday, today can be so much more valuable. We can appreciate the elemental joys of life—music, art, natural beauty, and poetry. Experiencing these joys allows for a deeper communication with our loved ones because, when we appreciate them, we are not caught up with the daily inconveniences of life.

Once we have faced death, there's not much that can scare us. What could we possibly be afraid of after having admitted to ourselves that we had dealt with the actual existence of our own mortality? Many who have battled cancer also have fewer interpersonal fears because they feel no one can ever have power over them again. It's very important not to see illness as a failure. This thinking arises out of viewing life as a competitive sport and dying as if it were the equivalent of losing. The truth is in this view, we are all losers eventually. It's easier said than done, but we must not focus on outcome, but rather on the joys we can find today. Unfortunately, too many people become deadened before they die. Interestingly, my cancer survivors experience much more gratitude than my "worried well" clients who still take their lives for granted. I'm reminded of the old joke about the two women who were on vacation in the mountains. One, complaining about the food, says, "It's horrible, tastes bad, looks bad," and the other says, "Yeah, and in such small portions." They seem to be saying that life is miserable and empty, but don't let this misery end.

Because we don't operate out of reality but rather our perception of reality, we can create a world in which gratitude is a significant factor. I have found the single biggest difference for a happy life and an unhappy life is the amount of gratitude that is felt. Happiness is not dependent on outward circumstances; healing is the result of a return to inner peace. Marcus Aurelius wrote in ancient times that the happiness of life depends on the quality of our thoughts. Keeping a journal, creating a joy biography and a gratitude log, enable us to contact that part of us that "knows it knows" so that when the body begins to heal, the spirit and the mind don't stay in intensive care. None of these thoughts are new. We can either come from faith or come from fear. It is our choice.

When our birth year and death year are listed, our time on this earth is symbolized by the dash between those years. How do you want to spend your dash? William Pukey suggests that you, "Dance like no one is watching, love like you'll never be hurt, sing like no one is listening, and live like it's heaven on earth."

CHAPTER NINETEEN

How to Get the Best Care and Treatment: Coordinated Breast Services and Physician Teams

By Claudia Z. Lee, M.B.A., and Ellen Tobin, M.ed.

As you may know from your own experience, facing a possible breast cancer diagnosis, or receiving a definitive diagnosis, creates a great deal of fear and anxiety, which can be compounded by not knowing what to do to find the best breast care. Even a well-informed person can become panicked after a diagnosis and feel obliged to make treatment decisions as quickly as possible. It is important to know that you have time.

Taking the time to research your options will not jeopardize your prognosis. For the most part, breast cancer treatment is not a medical emergency.[1] There is no need to rush into any decision. Two to three weeks will not make a difference in the clinical outcome of your treatment, yet taking the time to learn about your specific diagnosis[2] and treatment options can lead to a greater sense of control over and confidence in the treatment process. You have time to select physicians, and, if necessary, change them. Becoming a cancer patient is a new and diffi-

---

[1] The exceptions to this are inflammatory breast cancer and locally advanced disease.
[2] Breast cancer is not a single disease but rather a collection of many different types that may be in any of five different stages.

cult experience. You may be facing varied and unexpected emotions. You may not have had a serious health concern in the past, or you may not have dealt with other significant life crises. Deciding how to respond to this particular life event can be a challenge. You may or may not be accustomed to asserting yourself—that is, "taking charge" of a situation, finding information, insisting on the best care, and persisting until your needs are well met. This is definitely a time to consider moving from inaction—even if you are feeling temporarily overwhelmed— into action. Being assertive about your needs may help you to learn more about your disease, communicate effectively with your physicians, and get the level of care that you seek. However, we should state that each woman has the right to choose the approach that she will take to her own life-threatening illness. Some women want to be more involved in deciding the course of their treatment than do others.

Finding High-Quality Care Takes Effort

Every woman facing a breast cancer diagnosis wants state-of-the-art care. But many women with whom we have spoken have consistently said that they had no idea how difficult it was to obtain quality breast care—care that they trusted. One of the reasons for this is that our health care system is in fact not a system at all, but a blend of individual professionals and practices that tend to function more or less in isolation. Additionally, our health insurance system can be difficult to negotiate, often appearing to benefit insurers rather than patients. Even with good insurance, finding adequate health care can be a daunting task. When a woman has little or inadequate health care insurance, it can be even more difficult. For more information about potential resources for financial support, refer to the resource directory at the end of this book.

Most physicians are competent, caring professionals who want the best for their patients. Nevertheless, it is extremely difficult for them to remain current with all the important new information, recent research outcomes, and constantly evolving technology. We live in a world of information overload. Today's medical practices, therefore, are often highly specialized. This is certainly true for breast cancer diagnosis and treatment. Thus, you cannot assume that one physician will be just as adept at diagnosing or treating breast cancer as another, nor can you assume that your primary care physician will refer you to the most experienced clinicians to diagnose and treat your breast cancer. A recent Institute of Medicine study concluded that many cancer patients are not getting the care that cancer researchers know to be effective. In the past decade, there have been major advances in the treatment of breast cancer, some of them only within the past couple of years. As noted above, not every physician is well-informed on these changes. In other words, there is a disparity between ideal care and the everyday reality of treatment in various settings.[3] Although many organizations[4] have made quality improvement a high priority, there is still a need for diligence and careful attention to securing the very best care, as these organizations have suggested through their publications, their diagnostic/treatment guidelines, and their support of legislation, such as the Mammography Quality Standards Act (MQSA), which requires that mammography facilities meet certain standards in order to be accredited.

> Interdisciplinary team and comprehensive services for breast cancer patients are often organized into a breast cancer diagnosis and treatment program or a comprehensive breast center. Sometimes it is called a *breast program*. We use these terms interchangeably.

Finding and Evaluating an Interdisciplinary Breast Program

Many physicians and hospital staff have long been concerned that the needs of breast cancer patients were being inadequately met. When we ask patients about their experiences, we often hear stories that are dis-

---

[3] Institute of Medicine, 1999. "Ensuring Quality Cancer Care," Hewitt, M., Simone, J.V., Eds. Washington, D.C.: National Academy Press.

[4] The American College of Radiology (ACR), American Society of Clinical Pathologists, The Food and Drug Administration (FDA), the National Cancer Institute (NCI), the Association of Clinical Oncologists (ASCO), and the Agency for Healthcare Research and Quality (AHRQ).

turbing and indicative of a need to do more on the patients' behalf. We interviewed patients in focus groups, asking what they wanted in breast care. Their answers almost always mirrored the components of a good breast center. In this section, we will examine those attributes and help you find and assess a good breast cancer services program.

> *I was referred from one doctor to another. I was so worried that they weren't talking to each other about me that I carried my records including scans and mammograms with me every place I went. I kept them in my car so I wouldn't forget them. They (the doctors and the treatment staff) were all over the place, and I wasn't sure about any of them. I was my own case manager, my own nurse, my own educator, and my own everything. A breast center? It sounds wonderful! Lead me to it!*
>
> • Breast cancer patient in a focus group

To discuss the need for a biopsy, or after diagnosis of breast cancer has been made, many women typically make an appointment with a surgeon. But women often want to and should consult with other specialists early in the process as well, such as the radiation oncologist, if they are considering breast-saving surgery; the plastic surgeon, if they are considering a mastectomy with reconstruction; and the medical oncologist, whose expertise encompasses the use of chemotherapy and hormone therapy. (In some instances, chemotherapy may be given before surgery.) Also, as treatment progresses, they may seek opinions from a variety of medical professionals involved in their care. Breast cancer is a complex disease, requiring astute diagnosis, up-to-date treatment and skilled, compassionate support from health professionals in specialties that include radiology, pathology, breast surgery, radiation oncology, medical oncology, plastic surgery, nursing, psychology, and psychiatry. Ideally, we would like to see every woman who is facing a breast cancer diagnosis treated by an interdisciplinary breast care team that is associated with an organized comprehensive breast program. In such an interdisciplinary setting, you can be assured that physicians are working together on your behalf.

What Is a Comprehensive Breast Center or Program?

A comprehensive breast center is an organized delivery system in which all the medical and health professionals involved in the screening, diagnosis, treatment, and rehabilitation of breast cancer communicate so that you, the patient, can receive the benefit of their collaborative efforts. A breast center may be a physical site—for example, a facility with all services offered in one location—or it may be "virtual" with various services interacting with one another. The primary objective, however, is to make sure that each patient receives the highest level of care from physicians and other practitioners who are working together as a team. Quality care depends on coordinated services from expert practitioners.

If you do not have a breast program in your community, we suggest ways that you can achieve medical care with many of the same components as a breast program later in this chapter. It is more difficult, but possible.

Where Can You Find a Comprehensive Breast Program?

Breast centers are most likely to be found in or near hospitals (often in medical office buildings), including university and community hospitals, cancer centers, and women's centers. The number of breast programs has increased considerably over the last few years as women have become more informed about breast cancer and have begun to be more assertive in demanding patient-centered services that are timely, well-coordinated, and of high quality.

Breast centers are not necessarily organized to provide all services at the same time. Most physicians do not have their offices in the breast center, and there are excellent breast centers with no physician presence other than a clinical breast radiologist who is on-site when women with a breast concern are scheduled. Yet the center can still be arranged to reduce fragmentation of care and facilitate a team effort on behalf of each person with breast cancer. This is typically accomplished by the weekly treatment–planning breast conference and by the nurse naviga-tor. (See below.)

> *I want my doctors to work together on my behalf. I want advice at every juncture. I want my doctors to figure out what I don't know and then help me get the information I need. I don't want to be tracking down reports and reminding my doctors that I need an appointment with one of them. I also don't want to be wondering all the time if I have the best doctors and have selected the best treatment. I want someone to help me through this!* · Breast cancer patient in a focus group

How can you make sure that when you go to a "breast center" that the professional staff are all specialty trained in breast cancer diagnosis or care? It is not an easy task, but we will suggest a few questions to ask:

• **Do expert physicians who are experienced, well-trained, and dedicated to the diagnosis and treatment of breast cancer provide the care?** We will talk about this in detail later in this chapter. The most important clinical components of quality breast care include the breast radiologist and pathologist for diagnosis, and then the breast and plastic surgeons and the radiation and medical oncologists for treatment. However, the coordination of services that are typically part of a comprehensive breast program, including services that support your informational, emotional, nutritional, and social needs, is extremely important to your well-being. And this leads to the next important question.

• **Is there a nurse navigator, or coordinator, who facilitates the work-up and treatment decision processes, provides education and information based on patients' needs, and serves as a patient advocate?** When we ask cancer patients in focus groups about the first thing they want when they are newly diagnosed, they invariably answer, "I want a nice, smiling person to help me through this." Not all centers have such professionals. If you are assembling your own team or your breast center does not have a coordinator, ask

COMPONENTS OF A QUALITY COMPREHENSIVE BREAST CENTER

The following services represent a mature breast center that has been providing high-quality screening, diagnosis, and coordinated care for several years. Comprehensive does not necessarily mean "one-stop-shopping" with all the treatment modalities in the breast center, rather that there is an array of services, either on site or in the community that addresses the woman's emotional, informational, educational, and rehabilitative needs as well as mammography screening and diagnostic work-up to rule out or confirm breast cancer. These patient-centered breast programs have a focus on diagnostic timeliness, interdisciplinary collaboration, services coordination, and health care system navigation.

Screening and Diagnosis

Breast Imaging

- Radiologists and technologists who are subspecialized in breast imaging

- Dedicated, on-site breast ultrasound to facilitate resolution of the breast concern

- Timely imaging work-up of a breast problem

- Mammography Quality Standards Act (MQSA) accreditation that addresses personnel, equipment, and quality control.

Breast pathology

- Breast expertise in both cytopathology (cells) and histopathology (tissue)

- Meticulous approach to specimen acquisition, processing, margin, and tumor measurement

Interdisciplinary Treatment Planning

- Weekly discussion among all breast-related physician specialties to recommend appropriate treatment

- Adherence to widely accepted treatment guidelines

Emotional and Psychological Support

- Assessment, crisis intervention, and referral, if appropriate

- Assistance with navigating the health care system, such as making appointments and identifying resources

- Availability of support groups and trained breast cancer survivors with whom to speak

COMPONENTS OF A QUALITY COMPREHENSIVE BREAST CENTER
(*Continued*)

- Emotional support throughout the process from diagnosis through post-treatment, including extended survivorship

- Personal appearance center for wigs, prostheses, hats, scarves, and cosmetics

Education and Outreach
- Educational activities for patients, the community, and physicians

- Resource center with books, pamphlets, videos, and a computer for Internet searches, ideally including a health educator to help find relevant information

- Outreach activities to assist the medically underserved population, such as the elderly, special ethnic groups, and rural populations

Rehabilitation and Continuing Care
- Lymphedema program with well-trained therapists

- Risk assessment program including a multigenerational pedigree, appropriate lifestyle behavior counseling, and testing referral, if indicated

- Complementary medicine activities, such as tai chi, aqua aerobics, yoga, stretching, meditation, biofeedback, journaling, music and art therapy, as well as services such as nutrition and dietary education, information, and support. These programs are seldom housed in the center, but are usually nearby.

Research
- Availability of Phase III clinical trials within the community sponsored by large national cooperative research groups

- Referral to academic centers, NCI-designated comprehensive cancer centers, and the National Cancer Institute, for special studies and for Phase I and II trials, if appropriate

for an oncology nurse or a nurse who specializes in or is extremely knowledgeable about breast care. You are looking for someone who will walk you through the process, make sure you understand your treatment options, connect you with another breast cancer survivor, make certain you are seeing the right type of physician for the treatment you need (although nurses do not make direct referrals), and provide you with emotional support when necessary.

• **Does the breast center provide patient-focused, nonfragmented, and well-coordinated care by a compassionate and competent staff providing timely work-ups and easy access to services?** Even though the best breast centers in the country are experiencing long delays for mammography screening appointments, most breast centers make certain that there is a timely appointment for women who need breast imaging to rule out or confirm a breast problem. Likewise, if the symptomatic woman requires additional procedures such as ultrasound, the work-up is completed at that one appointment. If a biopsy is recommended, it is sometimes performed during the same visit, but it is usually scheduled for a few days later and may be provided by the breast radiologist or your surgeon.

• **Does the breast center offer the services of experienced breast radiologists rather than "general" radiologists?** A clinical breast radiologist is not merely a film reader, but rather a highly specialized breast-imaging consultant who directly interacts with symptomatic women and who works closely with the core team that includes both pathology and surgery. We will talk about this very important issue later in the chapter.

• **Do the physicians participate in weekly interdisciplinary treatment planning conferences?** Each week, physicians associated with a breast center meet to discuss newly diagnosed patients and those patients whose disease has recurred. The purpose of this interdisciplinary discussion is to reach a consensus treatment recommendation. We talk more about this later on as well.

• **What if my cancer recurs, will I still have the benefit of the weekly conference?** Absolutely. Breast cancer patients can be presented at the conference whenever there is a need for treatment planning.

• **Does the breast program have stage-specific breast cancer guidelines available for my review?** Most mature comprehensive breast programs use stage-specific breast cancer guidelines. These guidelines are evidence-based with all recommendations solidly backed by peer-reviewed research. The National Comprehensive Cancer Network (NCCN) has assembled expert panels to develop these guidelines for physicians. In conjunction with the American Cancer Society (ACS), NCCN also has developed comprehensive, user-friendly patient versions. You can obtain these breast cancer guidelines, free of charge, from either organization. For more information, see listings for the ACS and the NCCN in the resource directory.

• **Are supportive services available?** A diagnosis of breast cancer and its subsequent treatment frequently leads to emotional distress. Some patients need referrals to clergy, social workers, psychologists, or psychiatrists for additional help. Many patients benefit from support groups and specialized programs that carefully match breast cancer survivors with newly diagnosed patients. Sometimes busy health care professionals forget to ask about your emotional health. You may find it necessary to say, "I need a referral to a mental health professional" or "Please tell me about support groups."

• **What if I develop a swollen arm or hand?** Most communities have at least one lymphedema program with highly trained therapists who provide an extensive array of treatments and devices. Most breast centers provide lymphedema services, sometimes in collaboration with hospital rehabilitation departments. The National Lymphedema Network is an important resource. Please refer to the resource directory for their website.

• **Are education and outreach services available?** A quality breast program should offer on-site education and information resource centers, breast self-examination (BSE) training, as well as breast cancer community forums that are culturally sensitive. Assistance from a certified dietitian or nutritionist is also important for some patients.

• **Now that I have breast cancer, what are the risks to my family?** This is often one of the first questions newly diagnosed breast cancer patients ask. It is important to understand, however, that at this point in the genetic knowledge base 85 to 90 percent of breast cancer is considered "sporadic"—in other words, it is neither genetic nor hereditary. The issue of "risk" is extremely complicated. Many health care professionals, including physicians, do not have the genetics knowledge or experience in genetics to accurately counsel families of breast cancer patients. More and more breast centers are developing genetic risk counseling programs with professionals specifically trained in breast genetics. An excellent book written in lay language is *Assess Your True Risk of Breast Cancer* by Patricia Kelly, Ph.D.[5]

• **Does the breast center provide referrals?** Your program should provide referrals to any legitimate community or hospital resource that provides applicable breast services that are not provided at the breast center itself. These resources may include lymphedema rehabilitation, genetic risk assessment and counseling, psychological intervention, support groups, and complementary strategies, such as movement therapies (for example, tai chi and yoga), music therapy, and resources for spiritual guidance.

The Breast Cancer Team: Weekly Interdisciplinary Conferences Are a Key Part of Quality Care

Although you will have conferences with individual physicians in their offices, many breast center teams (physicians, nurses, geneticists, and mental health professionals) meet for pretreatment planning when a patient is diagnosed. The weekly interdisciplinary, prospective breast conference[6] is designed to address in part your concern about communication among physicians of every applicable specialty, but also to increase the knowledge base of every attendee and to assure that all treatment options are discussed.

---

[5] Kelly, Patricia T. *Assess Your True Risk of Breast Cancer.* New York: Henry Holt & Co., Owl Books, 2000.

[6] Lee, C. Z., "Interdisciplinary Weekly Prospective Breast Cancer Conference." *Journal of Oncology Management,* 3(6): 56–57, November/December, 1994.

After presentation of your individual breast cancer facts, the interdisciplinary breast team reaches a consensus recommendation about your treatment. This recommendation is usually shared with you by your surgeon. In addition to optimal therapies, there is discussion of potential research participation and family risk surveillance.

It is important to note that the conference does not dictate the treatment decision. The treatment decision is still your choice. But for many women, having their individual breast cancer cases discussed by the interdisciplinary physician team greatly increases their confidence in the entire process and in the selection of the physicians.

The authors' experience is that

> ## DOING YOUR HOMEWORK: RESOURCES FOR PHYSICIAN SELECTION
>
> You may wish to research information about your current or potential physicians on your own.
>
> The National Cancer Institute (NCI) developed The Physician's Data Query (PDQ) database to give physicians the latest information about cancer and cancer treatment. In addition to information about cancer care and available clinical trials, the NCI-PDQ database provides the names of hospitals and physicians involved in cancer care. You can check a physician's board certification, education (the institution at which your doctor did his or her residency is most important), teaching affiliations, publications (if any), and years of experience. You can access the database online or through a library with online searching capability.

this weekly prospective conference is one of the most beneficial programs offered as part of a comprehensive breast center. It is beneficial to the woman because she has the assurance that all her physicians are communicating and collaborating on her individual breast cancer and beneficial to the physicians because they have the assurance that each patient's breast cancer has the benefit of discussion by an interdisciplinary team of clinical peers.

The Treating Physicians: What to Expect, What to Ask

Whether a woman with breast cancer chooses treatment by physicians associated with a breast center or she carefully selects the medical consultants on her own, there are certain issues that are usually addressed. Often these issues are not quantifiable, such as a "personality fit" and "bedside manner," but they are very important to assess.

I think it's important to have a good rapport with the people who treat you, from your surgeon to the oncologist, who will follow you the rest of your life. It's important to feel comfortable and easy with them, to be able to talk to them. I have to say I had the best of everything, from biopsy onward. When I came in the office, they made me feel like a part of what was going on. • Linda R.

My doctor's staff was also especially helpful to me, handling problems with the insurance company and coordinating schedules between doctors. Of course, there is nothing to compare with the expertise and the fantastic bedside manner of my doctors. • Teresa

In addition to expertise, which we will discuss next, each of your doctors should share the following characteristics:

• Really "listen" and not merely hear.

• Describe breast cancer treatment options and the risks/benefits of each in understandable terms.

• Permit adequate time for the treatment decision.

• Encourage second opinions with a physician of the same discipline but from a different medical group.

• Ask about psychosocial issues including sexuality.[7]

• Support exploration on the Internet.

• Allow a tape recorder in the patient sessions.

• Be informed about complementary options that enhance patients' quality of life, be aware of the risk and benefits of herbal medicines and vitamins, and, in general, be open to complementary medicine discussions. This is particularly relevant to medical and radiation oncologists and nurses. Physicians may sometimes make a referral to a dietitian, a nutritionist, and/or other complementary medicine practitioners.

---

[7] Schain, W. S. "Physician-Patient Communication about Breast Cancer: A Challenge for the 1990s." *Surgical Clinics of North America*, 1990 (70): 917.

• Be accessible. Someone from the office should return your phone calls in a timely manner.

• Have a friendly, efficient staff. You will interact frequently with the staff members. They should be polite, informative, and compassionate.

Additional attributes to look for are the following:

• Board certification in their specialties.

• Active participation in weekly interdisciplinary, prospective breast conferences about each patient's care and treatment.

• Membership in specialty-specific professional organizations and ongoing participation in breast-specific seminars.

• Active medical staff privileges at the most respected hospital(s) in the area.

• Significant experience with procedures in his or her field. Ask your physician what percentage of his/her practice is devoted to breast cancer treatment.

Resources for Additional Questions to Ask

Many breast cancer organizations have lists of questions to facilitate discussion between patients and their physicians. These lists are free-of-charge and are available from the American Cancer Society, National Alliance of Breast Cancer Organizations (NABCO), the Susan G. Komen Breast Cancer Foundation, and the National Coalition for Cancer Survivorship, among many groups. See the resource directory at the end of this book for information.

The Physicians' Skills and Expertise

Many studies (including our own focus groups) indicate that most patients would rather go to physicians they already know and that primary care physicians often refer to physicians whom they see at their hospitals or whom they know socially. You want to make sure that you have selected the best breast expert. Nurses who work with breast physicians on a regular basis are often very helpful. Physicians who specialize in breast diagnosis and treatment will practice evidence-based medicine and consult practice guidelines that are developed based on evidence of successful outcomes. In other words, they will be active and current in breast cancer diagnosis and treatment.

The Radiologist

Breast imaging is usually the major procedural activity in a breast center. Over the last quarter of a century, breast imaging has become quite sophisticated in terms of technique, interpretation, and interventional procedures.[8] And, as demonstrated by the landmark Swedish study, mammography is the only radiologic procedure that directly impacts mortality[9] by actively searching for and finding early asymptomatic breast cancer that is curable if treated promptly and appropriately.

Does the Radiologist Who Is Interpreting the Mammograms and Performing the Breast Procedures Have a Vital Interest and Special Training in Breast Imaging?

High-quality breast centers in mid- to large-size urban areas have experienced clinical radiologists who subspecialize in breast imaging. These radiologists are responsible for all aspects of breast imaging: mammography, ultrasound, cyst aspiration, ductograms, and minimally invasive needle biopsies, which can be either ultrasound-guided or stereotactic-guided. Breast radiologists are members of the Society of Breast Imaging (SBI) and attend breast conferences every year.

In smaller communities, there may not be a breast imaging special-

---

[8] Sickles, E. A. "Breast Imaging: From 1965 to Present." *Radiology*, 2000 (215): 1–16.

[9] Tabar, I., Vitak, B., TonyChen, H. H., et al. "Beyond Randomized Controlled Trials: Organized Mammographic Screening Substantially Reduces Breast Carcinoma Mortality." *Cancer*, 2001, 91(9): 1724–1731.

ist, but there should be only a small number of radiologists (two to three) who interpret mammograms. If there are several "general" radiologists rotating through the breast center and if you have a symptom, you may want to request a second opinion on your mammogram.

The Pathologist

• What is the next step in the diagnostic process? The next step in the diagnostic process is the interpretation of breast tissue by the breast pathologist. Although pathology is not as visible in a breast center, the quality of the pathology is equally as important as the quality of the breast imaging. There are two subspecialties in breast pathology: cytopathology, which is the study of cells obtained by a skinny needle (that is, fine needle aspiration), and histopathology, which is the study of tissue obtained by a larger needle (that is, large core biopsy) or tissue obtained from a surgical biopsy. Breast cytopathologists are relatively rare in the United States and typically have their practices at academic centers or teaching hospitals. Most definitive breast biopsies in the community setting are tissue biopsies requiring the skills of a histopathologist.

• **Does the pathologist have special training and interest in breast pathology?** This is a critical question, because the details of the pathologist's diagnosis will influence your subsequent treatment. The meticulousness with which the pathologist obtains the tumor from surgery, processes the specimen (complete sequential sectioning for DCIS), measures the tumor, assesses the margins, and correlates the pathology findings with imaging and clinical findings is the degree to which you can be comfortable with the pathology report.[10] Unfortunately, it is very difficult for you to obtain all of this internal process-type information, but if the pathologist has a keen interest in breast pathology and regularly participates in and

---

[10] Lagios, M. D. "Pathology Procedures for Evaluation of the Specimen with Potential or Documented Ductal Carcinoma In Situ." *Seminars in Breast Disease,* 2000, 3(1): 42–49.

contributes to a breast center's weekly prospective breast conference, he or she has a higher likelihood of spending the extra time that is required for breast-specimen processing and interpretation. Your surgeon or pathologist will be able to answer your pathology-related questions.

• **How can the pathology report be translated into understandable terms?** Understanding your pathology report may be confusing, but the pathologist or surgeon will explain what each variable means. In addition, some books written for breast cancer patients describe the pathology report and what each section means.

• **Do the biopsy results make sense?** The most important issue is the correlation among the imaging findings, the pathology results, and the clinical findings, if any. You should ask for a copy of both the pathology report and radiology reports. Discuss these with your surgeon to make certain there is agreement among the findings. If there is not agreement, your breast concern has not been resolved, and you will need to continue the diagnostic work-up.

The Surgeon

The surgeon may be the first specialist you consult, or the second, depending on whether you had a diagnostic mammogram before your visit with the surgeon. When choosing your breast surgeon, you should be aware of the difference between a general surgeon who does many types of surgery and a specialist.[11] Although many surgeons perform breast surgery, the technology and techniques developed in recent years require additional training and new skills. There are many characteristics of an experienced breast surgeon. Breast surgery is becoming a specialized field. A significant amount of your surgeon's practice should be

---

[11] Hillner, B. E., Smith T. J., Desch, C. E. "Hospital and Physician Volume or Specialization and Outcomes in Cancer Treatment: Importance in Quality of Cancer Care." *Journal of Clinical Oncology,* 2000, 18(11): 2327–2340.

devoted to breast cancer surgery. Below are some other characteristics you want to look for:

• In many cases, the surgeon will refer you to the radiation oncologist, medical oncologist, or plastic surgeon prior to definitive surgery, depending on your particular situation. If not, ask the surgeon if these types of referrals are relevant to you preoperatively.

• The breast surgeon is skilled at breast-conserving surgeries (for example, lumpectomies) and supports that option over modified radical mastectomies unless there is a clinical, cosmetic, or patient choice reason for the mastectomy. For more information on breast-conserving surgery, see Chapter 6, "Saving the Breast."

• He or she will be experienced in performing newer techniques, such as skin-sparing procedures and sentinel lymph node biopsy. These and other techniques are discussed in other chapters.

• Breast surgeons are members of the American Society of Breast Surgeons (ASBS) and participate in their courses and other breast-specific seminars every year.

• He or she will work closely with a plastic surgeon to plan your surgery, if you are considering breast reconstruction. (See Chapter 9, "State-of-the-Art Breast Reconstruction.")

• The surgeon presents his or her newly diagnosed breast cancer patients to the weekly breast conference before the definitive surgery. Remember for 95 percent of the breast cancers, there is no need to rush surgery.

The Radiation Oncologist

If you have selected a breast center affiliated with a well-regarded hospital, you can usually be assured that the radiation oncologists and their equipment are of high quality. There is usually one radiation oncology group affiliated with a hospital, so you may want to concentrate on finding a radiation oncologist within that group with whom you are comfortable. In other words, you are looking for a good "personality fit." If you are assembling your own team, you will want to make sure that your radiation oncologist is highly regarded by your surgeon and that he or she is knowledgeable about and current on breast cancer radiation therapy. If you want to participate in radiation clinical trials, you will also want to ask your radiation oncologist if he or she enrolls patients in clinical trials sponsored by the Radiation Therapy Oncology Group (RTOG) or any of the clinical research cooperative groups.

The Medical Oncologist

Your medical oncologist is the physician who evaluates the necessity for and prescribes systemic treatments, such as chemotherapy and hormone therapy. For many patients, the medical oncologist is the primary physician for cancer care after surgery and radiation. Your medical oncologist will see you through care, provide treatment, and monitor your condition after treatment. That is why it is important that your oncologic physicians keep your primary care physician informed of your treatment and disease status. Look for the following characteristics when selecting your medical oncologist:

• He or she will be an active member of the Association of Clinical Oncologists (ASCO) and attend their conferences.

• He or she usually has access to clinical trials.[12] Many patients we have interviewed do not understand how important it is to be in a location where research is valued. Clinical trials may or may not be appropriate for you. Even if you do not participate in a clinical trial, you will want to know that your oncologist has access to

---

12 The National Surgical Adjuvant Breast and Bowel Project (NSABP) conducts clinical research in many cancer centers and physician offices. Other cooperative groups are Southwestern Oncology Group (SWOG), the Eastern Cooperative Oncology Group (ECOG), and the Radiation Therapy Oncology Group (RTOG). Check the NCI listing in the resource directory for links to the trials sponsored by these organizations.

state-of-the-art clinical research, either conducting the research through his or her practice or referring to other centers, if appropriate. You may want to seek clinical trial information from the Internet (see the resource directory at the end of this book) and ask your physicians about a trial's applicability to your specific situation.

• The medical oncologist will support the use of newer treatments to reduce symptoms and side effects of chemotherapy, such as fatigue, nausea, pain, or other discomfort. He or she will be familiar with the use of hormones that stimulate blood cell growth and reduce the degree of suppression of blood cell counts after chemotherapy. For information, see Chapter 10, "Chemotherapy, Hormone Therapy, and the Stages of Breast Cancer."

• Your oncologist will discuss the risks and benefits of different types of therapies. He or she should also provide you with a hopeful, but realistic prognosis. If your prognosis does not point to long-term survival, your medical oncologist should assure you of the availability of "comfort" or palliative care that relieves symptoms and enhances quality of life in the event that aggressive treatment is not likely to be helpful.

The Internist, Gynecologist, and Family Physician

These physicians are absolutely critical in the breast care continuum. They must be very knowledgeable about signs and symptoms, risk factors, hormone replacement, clinical breast exams, and other issues related to breast cancer. They must be astute when listening to women in order to identify subtle breast concerns women may be afraid to state. They work in close partnership with patients and with the diagnostic and treatment team. Your primary physician is the one constant link within the entire breast cancer process. Ultimately, you will return to your primary physician after treatment. In fact, in some managed care situations, the primary physician monitors you beginning one year after treatment. If you do not have a primary physician, it is imperative that you find one.

Write all your questions down. Ask anything, even if it's silly. If you are not happy with the answers you receive or if you are not getting answers, seek a second opinion. Find a doctor you can talk to. Go to a support group. They help, they really do. • Cynthia

Be an aware consumer. If you are not happy with the advice you are given, find someone else who can help you. Knowledge is power. Find answers to your questions. • Anne

Ask anything you think you should know. We've grown up thinking that doctors know everything. But it's our responsibility to gather information and to know what the options are. All my doctors were more than willing to answer questions, and I think that's key. • Linda R.

Navigating the System

Once you have determined the qualities you seek in a breast cancer center or program and the characteristics, skills, and experience you require of your physicians, you will begin the search for quality care in your community. How does one go about obtaining recommendations for physicians and other professionals?

• **Ask your primary care physicians, friends, associates, clergy, and especially physicians and nurses.** Check with local hospitals or those on your insurance list. Look at the Web site of the National Consortium of Breast Centers.[13] Check the Web site of the American College of Surgeons (www.facs.org) to make sure that your hospital has a cancer program that has earned Commission on Cancer approval. Call various breast centers in your community and ask to speak with the coordinator or the nurse in charge. Take your time. It will not hurt your prognosis.

---

[13] National Consortium of Breast Centers (www.breastcare.org) is a membership organization. It does not serve as an accreditation organization. Some breast centers listed are not comprehensive breast centers. Some very good breast centers are not members, especially those at academic facilities. Also, listings do not always have up-to-date information. Nevertheless, it can be a starting point. Centers are listed by state.

When my gynecologist found a lump, he referred me to a surgeon. I went to him, and he ordered a mammogram and then he did a biopsy. They said I needed a mastec-tomy. Somebody I work with said, "Why don't you get another opin-

> It may be that you are able to find an excellent breast center or well-coordinated services. Or, it may be that you need to develop your own team. Regardless of what approach you take, you will still need certain navigational assistance.

ion?" She referred me to a nurse friend who coordinated a referral to a surgeon. The second surgeon reviewed my mammogram and my pathol-ogy. I had an extremely small tumor, and the doctors had a conference. They recommended a lumpectomy. I had radiation and lots of support from the team. • Breast cancer patient in a focus group

• **Get a second opinion.** Ask your own physician for a referral for a second opinion, preferably at another center—perhaps at an ACoS-approved cancer program in a community hospital,[14] an academic center, or one of the NCI-designated cancer centers.[15] This would be an excellent opportunity to have the pathology slides or reports reviewed as well, particularly, if you select an NCI cancer center. Most physicians encourage second opinions, but if your physician(s) feel threatened by this action, you might want to consider changing physicians. If you want to initiate your own second opinion, call the leading hospital's central appointment number or check their website.

In what other ways can I increase my sense of security within the complex health care system?

• **Identify your nurse-navigator.** As we mentioned, most organ-ized breast programs will have a nurse-coordinator to help you dur-ing the entire work-up and decision-making and treatment process. If not, you will want to identify an oncology nurse who can help you arrange all aspects of your care.

---

[14] The Commission on Cancer of the American College of Surgeons (ACoS) has granted approval to cancer programs in 1,431 hospitals at the time of this writing. Most programs are community based.
[15] The National Cancer Institute has designated 60 cancer centers meeting criteria for research, teaching, and clinical care.

• **Communicate with your physicians**. Some physicians have less than ideal bedside manners while others are actually trained in "breaking bad news." Skilled physicians carefully assess each woman's personal and clinical situation, clearly describe all the appropriate treatment options, and provide hope and empathy. Come armed with your questions. Keep them short and to the point. Consider using a tape recorder. If at all possible, bring someone to listen and take notes. During this time of great stress, you may have difficulty remembering the details of the discussion.

• **Obtain additional information**. Although your physician will describe your treatment options to you, many women want to read additional material so that they clearly understand the issues. It is very helpful to obtain written information such as the NCCN/ACS breast cancer guidelines for patients. As soon as possible, find out the stage and type of your breast cancer (determined after the biopsy and through your pathology analysis) so that you can better evaluate your choices. Although you will have help making the treatment decision, it is your responsibility to know as much as possible about your disease, its treatment, and the potential side effects so that the decision is, in fact, an informed decision. Think about the trade-off for each treatment option. For example, some treatments give a statistically insignificant edge but may have long-lasting side effects that can greatly affect your quality of life. Do not think you are a coward if you do not opt for the most aggressive treatment.

• **Seek information from the National Cancer Institute** through their website or with one of their knowledgeable health educators (1-800-4-CANCER or one of the breast cancer websites). We have provided a list of websites that will help in the resource directory at the end of this book. It is important to note that not all websites are equally valuable or correct. Unfortunately, some websites are taking advantage of frightened cancer patients and suggesting treatment that is not only unproven but also harmful. Some are even selling "medicine." Seek information only from those websites that are supported by high-quality cancer centers, professional organizations, and well-known advocacy groups, such as the Susan G. Komen Breast Cancer Foundation, The National Alliance of Breast Cancer

GETTING THROUGH TREATMENT

Here are some things you can do to help yourself get through the treatment process:

- Keep your physician informed of any herbal or vitamin treatment you are taking or considering taking. Some supplements need to be stopped prior to surgery and some change the way chemotherapy and other drugs interact with your body.

- Make sure you get good explanations of what will happen before, during, and after radiation and chemotherapy.

- If you have fever, pain, nausea, extreme fatigue, or other symptoms, notify your doctor immediately.

- Ask yourself, are you exhausted, nauseated, not eating, depressed? If so, help is available through pharmaceutical intervention, "talking" interventions, and/or sometimes through behavior and lifestyle changes.

- Take special care during your "nadir," which is the time when your resistance is especially low because of the effects of chemotherapy on your bone marrow. Stay out of crowds and, if possible, away from children. Ask your physician if there is a need to boost either your white or red cells through medication

- Practice self-care. Eat as well as you can. Take supportive medications as suggested by your physician. Exercise and do movement therapies. Consider an "endorphin team." Later in this chapter we will introduce you to the idea of an endorphin team and help you put one together.

Organizations, The National Coalition for Cancer Survivorship, Y-ME, and Cancer Care, Inc. It is important to be Internet-savvy, but do not come into your physician's office with reams of articles. Instead, bring a paragraph or two, or a citation, and assume that your doctor will have read it.

• **Keep copies of your own records**. Even the most efficient office can lose records. Unless you are in a comprehensive center, especially one with computerized records, your records are likely to be in the office of the physician you last visited. When you are assured that this loss is not likely to occur, you can relax. On the other hand, you may want to keep a copy of your current records, such as reports on your CT scans and most recent blood work, so that you can refer to them in discussions with medical professionals.

Until I was comfortable that my physicians' offices would not lose my records, I kept the scans, X rays, and reports with me. When I go for a second opinion, I carry everything with me, including my physician's note. • Ellen

Being Your Own Advocate: A Checklist

For many women, the most satisfactory physician relationship is based on mutual respect, where the physician involves the woman in the decision-making process, is not paternalistic, and acknowledges that she is an intelligent being capable of understanding new information and asking relevant questions. In order to encourage this positive working relationship with your physician, the following tactics may be helpful:

• Be on time to your appointment. Unless you are really sick, dress as if you are going to work. It will put you in a better frame of mind and help you to feel confident in your interactions with your physician.

• Realize that the members of the nursing, clerical, and medical staff can be some of your best advocates. Treat them respectfully. They have very difficult responsibilities and tend to respond better to people who are upbeat. Smile, make little jokes, ask about their children, say "thank you" for good care. If you have treated staff members well, they will be there for you on your bad days. If you are someone who complains all the time, it is may be difficult for the staff to distinguish a genuine complaint from a habitual complaint. However, if you complain infrequently, you are likely to get an immediate and helpful response when you do express your concern.

• Tears are perfectly acceptable. Hugs are likely to be forthcoming if you want them. You may have to assert yourself to make sure your needs are known, but it is important to consider the staff's position as well and to be judicious about when to become insistent.

• Do not call the physician more than is absolutely necessary. Often the nurse can answer your questions or ask the physician on your behalf. Some physicians are comfortable sharing their email address and others are not. If you do have your physician's email address, it is important that you contact him or her only when necessary.

• In urgent situations, however, always have the appropriate phone numbers on hand and call them immediately.

• Medicine is an art as well as a science. For most breast centers, the NCCN guidelines will be followed, but sometimes there are very valid clinical, cosmetic, or psychological reasons why your physician recommends deviating from those guidelines. The important issue is that the physician clearly describes why a particular treatment is being recommended and that all of the options have been discussed by the interdisciplinary breast team.

• In most cases, you should not expect to attend the treatment planning meetings. It is very difficult for physicians to openly discuss and debate clinical issues related to your case if you are present. Be assured that your physician will promptly notify you of the conference outcome.

• If there is not an interdisciplinary breast center team that communicates and collaborates on a formal and regular basis, you may want to directly tell your physician that you want him or her to be the "captain of your team" and that you want him or her to specifically speak to Drs. X, Y, and Z.

In summary, the diagnosis and treatment of breast cancer has become quite subspecialized. This chapter is intended for those women who want to be fully informed about their breast cancer and to be active in their treatment decision-making. We have suggested several ways to maximize the likelihood that you will receive timely, coordinated, quality care.

| CARING FOR YOURSELF: THE ENDORPHIN TEAM

You will find a lot of useful information about caring for yourself in this book. Take a look at Chapter 17, "Your Emotions after Breast Cancer: Detecting Depression," even if you are not depressed, and Chapter 18, "Becoming Strong at the Broken Places." You will also read helpful advice from the breast cancer survivors who generously offered their comments to this book. I am also a cancer survivor and I want to share with you the way in which I was able to care for myself during treatment and to pass along the idea of the "endorphin team" to others.

When I was diagnosed with cancer, my world went into a tailspin. Like other cancer patients, I was terrified, depressed, and confused. To further compound the problem, I experienced feelings of social isolation. I was used to being active and in control. Now I sat around most of the time, except for visits to the doctor. My busy professional life came to a standstill. My family tried to console me, but I needed more. To my surprise and with my everlasting gratitude, my friends, family, and colleagues went into action. And they did it in a dramatic and powerful way. Some lived far away but they gave me what I needed: love and support. They each took a role, mostly unplanned, I think. One colleague taught me how to use the Internet, several professional colleagues gave me information about treatment and how to manage side effects, others provided medical contacts, and my colleagues kept me in the loop professionally. Some friends prayed for me. Amazingly, some people I barely knew came forward and corresponded with me. The conduit for most of this dialogue was email. I printed all the emails and filed them away for "rainy days."

Most of all, they made me laugh. A male friend wore a blond wig to visit me in chemotherapy. Several friends sent really awful jokes. I got cheerful but funny notes, telephone calls, and visits. My friends and relatives recognized that humor is my way of dealing with difficult situations. I decided that they were my endorphin team.

Endorphins, according to the dictionary are ". . . hormones with painkilling and tranquilizing ability that are secreted by the brain." Laughing and exercise stimulate endorphins. When I recovered, I tried to determine the properties of my endorphin team and how other patients could use it. In the meantime, in search of systematizing the process, I helped others set up a support system for members of our synagogue who may have needs similar to mine. We call it *Chizuk*, which means support or strength in Hebrew. The attributes are similar to my endorphin team but because we all live near to each other, we have added food to the mix—humor, socializing, and food mix well! We have also added a "captain" who helps to organize friends on the team. For some, we have also included prayer and study.

CARING FOR YOURSELF: THE ENDORPHIN TEAM
(*Continued*)

Rules of endorphin teams:

- "Recruit" your own team members by telling people about your situation.

- Ask for specific types of help. Remember that it makes people feel good to be helpful.

- Ask for correspondence.

- Thank everyone; tell them how much you appreciate their thoughtfulness.

- When you are well, return the favor.

- Reassemble the team whenever necessary.

- Include family members on your endorphin team.

- Accept the fact that some people will be frightened and may turn away. If you value their friendship, do not let them go without an effort to involve them.

- Try not to have negative (toxic) people around you.

BREAST CANCER RESOURCES

The American Cancer Society (ACS)
1-800-ACS-2345
http://www.cancer.org
The ACS is a nationwide, community-based voluntary health organization dedicated to eliminating cancer as a major health problem. Patient service programs are available throughout the country. The following may be available in your community: Look Good . . . Feel Better, which helps women learn to overcome the appearance-related side effects of cancer treatment and Reach to Recovery, which offers one-on-one visitation for women who have concerns about breast cancer. Also access The National Cancer Information Center, where trained cancer information specialists are available 24 hours a day, seven days a week to answer questions on cancer and link callers to resources in their communities.

Breast Cancer.Net
http://www.breastcancer.net/bcn.html
Articles on breast cancer and treatment as well as information on cancer centers and support groups.

BreastLink
http://www.breastlink.org
Provided by the Breast Cancer Care and Research Fund, this site offers articles on breast cancer, resources, and news.

Cancer Care, Inc.
1-800-813-HOPE (4673)
http://www.cancercare.org

Cancer Care is a nonprofit organization whose mission is to provide free professional help to people with all cancers through counseling, education, information and referral, and direct hotline assistance. Cancer Care has a staff of professional oncology social workers that can provide emotional support, assistance in coping with treatment and treatment side effects, and help talking to your doctor or other health care providers. Services are available through email, the above toll-free number, or in person. Educational seminars, teleconferences, professionally led support groups, information about cancer and treatment, and resources finding financial assistance are also available as are extensive links online to resources that include coping with treatment side effects, where to go for support, complementary and alternative treatments, breast cancer advocacy, breast cancer books, medical information about breast cancer, male breast cancer, advanced breast cancer, state Pharmaceutical Assistance Programs, mammography and detection, Medication Manufacturer's Indigent Drug Programs, finding financial assistance, finding home care, hospice care, and patient-to-patient networks.

Susan G. Komen Breast Cancer Foundation
1-800-I'M-AWARE or 1-800-462-9273
http://www.breastcancerinfo.com/bhealth/

Among its many other activities, the Susan G. Komen Breast Cancer Foundation offers information on breast cancer, risk factors, early detection, diagnosis and staging, living with breast cancer, support groups, and information for special populations.

National Black Women's Health Project (NBWHP)
http://www.nationalblackwomenshealthproject.org/

NBWHP seeks to improve the health of black women by providing wellness education and services, health information, and advocacy. Search articles on breast cancer, news, and links.

The National Consortium of Breast Centers, Inc. (NCBC)
http://www.breastcare.org

The mission of The National Consortium of Breast Centers, Inc., is "to promote excellence in breast health care for the general public through a network of diverse professionals dedicated to the active exchange of ideas and resources." Search the directory of breast centers, breast professionals, and clinical trials.

National Alliance of Breast Cancer Organizations (NABCO)
1-888-80-NABCO
http://www.nabco.org
1-212-719-0154
NABCO offers information, resources, and referrals to patients, survivors, and professionals and works to promote regulatory change and legislation that benefits survivors and women at risk. Search the site for basic facts and statistics on cancer, support groups nationwide, information for people recently diagnosed, and information about recurrent and advanced breast cancer.

National Coalition for Cancer Survivorship (NCCS)
1-301-650-9127 or 1-877-NCCS-YES (1-877-622-7937)
http://www.cansearch.org
NCCS is a national advocacy organization. Its website contains information about survivorship programs, links to websites, news, and information about conferences and events. Information available in Spanish.

The National Comprehensive Cancer Network (NCCN)
1-888-909-NCCN
http://www.nccn.org
NCCN is a not-for-profit alliance of the world's leading cancer centers. Developed in conjunction with the American Cancer Society (ACS), patient versions of practice guidelines can be downloaded or requested by mail.

National Lymphedema Network (NLN)
1-800-541-3259
http://www.lymphnet.org
NLN is an internationally recognized nonprofit organization founded to provide education and guidance to lymphedema patients, health care professionals, and the general public by disseminating information on the prevention and management of primary and secondary lymphedema. Services include referrals to lymphedema treatment centers, health care professionals, training programs, and support groups, among other resources.

OncoLink
University of Pennsylvania Cancer Center
http://www.oncolink.upenn.edu/disease/breast
This site offers an overview of breast cancer and information about types of breast cancer, treatment options, coping with cancer, clinical trials, cancer resources, support, and news.

Sisters Network
http://www.sistersnetworkinc.org/
Resources for African-American breast cancer survivors include lists of meetings and locations, connection with another woman on a message board, cancer facts, education, news, and events.

Y-ME Breast Cancer Organization
24-hour Y-ME National Breast Cancer Hotlines
1-800-221-2141 (English) or 1-800-986-9505 (Spanish)
http://www.y-me.org/
The mission of Y-ME National Breast Cancer Organization is to decrease the impact of breast cancer, create and increase breast cancer awareness, and ensure, through information, empowerment, and peer support, that no one faces breast cancer alone. Staffed largely by breast cancer survivors, Y-ME is a national organization with affiliate partners in 27 cities across the country. The website contains information about breast cancer and treatment options, resource links, a listing of support groups, publications, suggestions for talking with your family about breast cancer, and more.

The U.S. National Cancer Institute
1-800-4-CANCER
http://www.cancer.gov/
A division of the National Institutes of Health (NIH), the NCI has a hotline and a large website to help cancer patients with a variety of issues, including physician referrals, lists of NCI-designated cancer centers, clinical trials, statements on various cancer diagnoses, and booklets about cancer treatment and care. There are patient and physician versions. The physicians' information is part of PDQ (Physicians' Data Query) and is available to patients.

LITERATURE SEARCHES

How to Research Medical Literature
http://cancerguide.org/research. html
Explains how to use databases and online resources and links to other sources of helpful information on researching medical literature.

How to Read a Medical Paper—*British Medical Journal*
http://darkwing.uoregon.edu/~jbonine/howtoread.html
Contains information on how to read medical papers.

National Breast Cancer Awareness Month

http://www.nbcam.org/

Topics covered include finding information on breast cancer, treatment options, clinical trials, genetic testing, financial assistance, getting a quality mammogram, and support groups, among others. Some information in Spanish.

National Library of Medicine

http://www.ncbi.nlm.nih.gov/PubMed

Search PubMed located at the National Institutes of Health (NIH). Access citations and links to full-text journal articles.

BREAST CANCER GENETICS

GeneClinics™

http://www.geneclinics.org

Funded by the National Institutes of Health (NIH) and developed at the University of Washington, Seattle, GeneClinics™ provides health care practitioners and patients with current, authoritative information on genetic testing. The website contains a directory of clinics.

CLINICAL TRIALS

(Also see Cancer Care, the Susan G. Komen Breast Cancer Foundation, NABCO, and OncoLink above.)

ClinicalTrials.gov

http://www.clinicaltrials.gov/

Developed by the National Institutes of Health (NIH) through the National Library of Medicine, ClinicalTrials.gov provides information about clinical research studies. Search clinical trials by specific information and links to resource information, including MEDLINE*plus*, NIH Health Information, and Healthfinder®.

HopeLink

http://www.hopelink.com

Includes a directory of clinical trials open for enrollment.

CANCER AND THE ENVIRONMENT

Center for Bioenvironmental Research (CBR)

At Tulane and Xavier Universities

http://www.cbr.tulane.edu

Among its other activities, the Center for Bioenvironmental Research (CBR) at Tulane and Xavier universities has developed a holistic research program for disease prevention in humans and ecosystems. Search the website for information about environmental toxins and related information.

GLOSSARY

Adenocarcinoma: cancer that occurs in the glandular tissues. Most breast cancers are adenocarcinomas.

Adjuvant therapy: treatments given in addition to local treatment (such as surgery and radiation), for example, chemotherapy and hormone manipulation therapy

Adriamycin: a chemotherapy drug.

Anti-angiogeneis agents: drugs that block the formation of new blood vessels that are essential for tumor growth.

Antibody: a protein made by the immune system that recognizes and fights foreign substances in the body.

Antidepressants: drugs used to treat depression.

Antiemetics: medication that reduces nausea and vomiting that may result from chemotherapy. Examples of newer antiemetics are Zofran and Anzemet.

Antiestrogen: a hormone that acts to block the action of estrogen.

Anxiolytic: an antianxiety drug, such as Xanax or Valium.

Areola: the dark skin surrounding the nipple.

Aromatase inhibitors: drugs that stop the synthesis of estrogen from the ovaries and adrenal glands. Aromatase inhibitors have only been shown to be effective in women after menopause; but in postmenopausal women, aromatase inhibitors appear to be equal to and possibly better than tamoxifen in metastatic breast cancer.

Atypia: cells that have early changes that could develop into cancer or cells that are near cancer cells.

Atypical ductal hyperplasia (ADH): cells that increase the risk of developing cancer.

Axilla: the region in the armpit where many of the lymph nodes are found.

Axillary node dissection: surgical removal of a number of lymph nodes.

Beta-glucoronidase: a bacterial enzyme in the intestines.

Bilateral mastectomy: removal of both breasts.

Bracketing wire localization: a procedure in which the radiologist uses localization needles to place two or more wires into the breast around the edge of a suspected or documented cancer preoperatively using either mammographic, ultrasound, or stereotactic guidance. This procedure is done to allow the surgeon to attempt complete removal of a nonpalpable tumor without directly contacting it.

Breast-ovary cancer syndrome: an inherited mutation in one of the two copies of either the gene BRCA-1 or BRCA-2.

Breast-saving surgery: surgery for breast cancer that preserves the breast. These include lumpectomy (also called *wide excision* or *partial mastectomy*) and quadrantectomy.

Breast-skin erythema: redness of the breast skin.

Capsular contracture: tightening of breast tissue around a breast implant.

Central duct excision: an outpatient procedure in which a breast duct is removed through a small incision at the edge of or within the areola.

Central quadrantectomy: a quadrantectomy that includes the nipple and areola.

Chemotherapy: regimen of drugs used to kill cancer cells.

Clear margin: a rim of normal tissue—that is, tissue without cancer cells—between the cancer and the edge of the lumpectomy.

Coenzyme Q10: an antioxidant.

Core needle biopsy: a type of needle biopsy in which a needle is used to collect a sliver of tissue from a breast abnormality for diagnosis. Core needle biopsies may be done by hand, ultrasound, or stereotactic mammographic guidance.

Cosmetic quadrantectomy: removal of approximately a quarter of the breast with a simultaneous attempt to clear the margins of a larger breast cancer. This can be done with a flap advancement procedure to minimize any dipping or caving of the breast postoperatively.

Coumadin: a blood thinner.

CT (or CAT) scan: computerized tomography scan, a computer controlled X-ray system that can take cross-sectional images of a part of the body.

Cyclophosfamide (Cytoxan): a chemotherapy drug.

Cyst: a sac filled with fluid. Some breast cysts have a growth on the inner wall or solid material inside. These are called *complex cysts*.

Cytology: the study of individual and groups of cells.

Cytopathology: the study of cellular changes as they relate to disease.

Diagnostic mammogram: directed mammography used to aid in the diagnosis of an abnormality detected on a screening mammogram. The two most common views are magnification and spot compression, in which breast tissue is displaced using a compression paddle that is smaller than the one used with a standard mammogram.

Digital mammogram: a type of mammogram that uses digital imagery and computer analysis to aid in the interpretation of mammograms.

Docetaxel: a chemotherapy drug.

Doxorubicin (Adriamycin): a chemotherapy drug.

Ductal carcinoma in situ (DCIS): preinvasive breast cancer in which cancer cells have not yet traveled outside the ducts that carry milk to the nipple.

Ductal lavage: a technique of analyzing cells inside breast ducts by washing the cells out with fluid through the nipple.

Duct ectasia: a condition in which the ducts behind the nipple are inflamed and dilated, which can cause nipple discharge.

Ductogram: a test to detect a growth or tumor behind the nipple when a woman has a brown or bloody nipple discharge. This is done with a mammogram and a tiny catheter inserted into the nipple that injects dye into the discharging duct.

Ductoscopy: a technique of looking into breast ducts using tiny endoscopes inserted through small openings in the nipple.

Edema: swelling.

Electrocautery: an electrical surgical tool used to coagulate blood vessels and divide tissue.

Erythropoietin (Procrit or Epogen): a hormone that stimulates red blood cells used to improve anemia and reduce transfusions in people receiving chemotherapy.

Estradiol: the most active form of estrogen.

Estrogen (and progesterone) hormone receptors: surface proteins on breast cancer cells to which estrogen and progesterone can bind to promote cell division.

Excisional biopsy: simple removal of a small lump or nodule with no attention to microscopic margins.

False positive: a test result that indicates the presence of disease when there is no disease. A false negative test result indicates no disease when there is disease.

Fibroadenoma: a benign round lump that moves easily within the breast.

Fibrocystic breast: lumpiness in the breast, which can be accompanied by pain and tenderness, especially before the menstrual cycle.

Fine needle aspiration: a type of biopsy in which a very thin needle is used to withdraw cells for microscopic evaluation.

Flap advancement: a local surgical procedure done in concert with larger lumpectomies and quadrantectomies that frees up and reapproximates the back edges of the breast, allowing for better cosmetic results by minimizing dipping and caving of the breast postoperatively.

Flap reconstruction: a type of breast reconstruction done with your own tissues brought in from another area of the body.

Focal density: a dense area on a mammogram that cannot be defined as a mass, but may have the potential to be one.

Follicle-stimulating hormone: a pituitary hormone involved in the menstrual cycle and the production of estrogen and progesterone.

Free radicals: reactive oxygen molecules that can destroy cells.

Frozen section diagnosis: a microscopic evaluation of the specimen surgically removed from your breast performed while you are on the operating table under anesthesia.

Genistein: an isoflavone compound found in soy.

Hematopoietic cytokines: special hormones that stimulate blood cell growth.

Hemocult test: a test for microscopic amounts of blood.

Heparin: a blood thinner.

Her2/neu: a gene that makes a protein product that is on the surface of the cell and sometimes present in excess amounts on breast cancer cells.

Herceptin: a designer antibody shown to be effective in targeting cells that make too much her2/neu.

Histologic grade: the microscopic evaluation of a cancer type and structure.

Histology: the study of tissues.

Hormone replacement therapy: use of the hormones estrogen and progesterone from plant or animal sources to treat difficulties associated with menopause.

Image-guided biopsy: needle biopsies that are done for nonpalpable lesions with imaging techniques such as ultrasound and stereotactic mammographic guidance.

Immunohistochemical (IHC) staining: a method of evaluating lymph nodes for the presence of cancer using monoclonal antibodies, which can target specific proteins produced by cancer cells.

Implant reconstruction: reconstruction of the breast after mastectomy using a tissue expander device or a saline or silicone implant.

Indole-3-carbinol (I3C): a phytochemical obtained from cruciferous vegetables.

Inflammatory breast cancer: a rare, aggressive type of breast cancer that causes redness of the breast skin.

Insulin: a hormone that brings glucose into the cells to use as a fuel source.

Interleukin 2 (Neumega): a naturally occurring chemical in the body that increases the number of platelets, which helps prevent bleeding. Interleukin 2 acts by increasing levels of thrombopoietin, another naturally occurring body chemical that directly stimulates bone marrow cells to make more platelets.

Internal mammary nodes: lymph nodes behind the ribs near the sternum (breastbone).

Intraductal papilloma: a small benign growth in the breast duct, which can cause a bloody nipple discharge.

Intra-mammary lymph nodes: lymph nodes located inside the breast.

Lactating adenomas: a benign solid tumor in the breast that can occur during lactation.

Latissimus dorsi myocutaneous flap: surgery employing the latissimus dorsi muscle, skin, and fat from the back to reconstruct the breast after mastectomy or quadrantectomy.

Lesion: an area of abnormality.

Lobular carcinoma in situ (LCIS): a pre-cancer confined to the lobules where milk is produced in the breast, which increases the lifetime risk of breast cancer.

Local recurrence: recurrence of cancer in the breast or the immediate chest wall area.

Local treatment: treatment of the tumor in the breast, as with surgery and radiation.

Lumpectomy (also called wide excision or partial mastectomy): removal of a solid or radiographic tumor with a simultaneous attempt to clear the margins of suspected or documented breast cancer.

Luteinizing hormone: a pituitary hormone that stimulates the ovary during the menstrual cycle.

Lymphedema: swelling in the soft tissues of the arm and/or chest wall.

Lymph nodes: small glands that are part of your immune system and help protect you from bacteria, viruses, and other microorganisms.

Mammotome (also called directed vacuum-assisted biopsy): a type of core needle biopsy that employs a vacuum canister to pull breast tissue into the needle for biopsy. This type of biopsy is particularly useful for microcalcifications.

Margin of clearance: the least amount of normal breast tissue between the edge of the cancer and the edge of the lumpectomy. Getting a clean margin—that is, a clear rim of normal tissue—is critical to controlling the recurrence of a tumor in the breast.

Mastectomy: surgical removal of the breast.

> **Modified radical mastectomy:** removal of the breast without the chest wall muscles with appropriate axillary lymph node sampling.

> **Radical mastectomy:** removal of the major and minor chest wall muscles. This type of surgery is rarely done today.

> **Skin-sparing mastectomy:** removal of the breast with a minimal amount of skin necessary to effectively clear the margins. This is performed with immediate reconstruction.

> **Simple mastectomy:** removal of the breast without removal of the lymph nodes.

Mastitis: infection of the breast.

Mastopexy: a breast lift.

Medical oncologist: a physician who specializes in the medical treatment of cancer.

Megakaryocyte growth development factor (MGDF): a modified version of thrombopoietin that stimulates an increase in platelet numbers.

Metabolite: a product of metabolism.

Microcalcifications: tiny flecks of calcium in the breast visible on a mammogram. They are usually benign, but can indicate DCIS, especially when they are tightly clustered.

Milk cysts: a cyst full of milk that can occur during lactation.

Monoclonal antibodies: designer antibodies, created in the laboratory, that target specific markers on or in tumor cells. Some monoclonal antibodies are used by pathologists to study tumor specimens and others are used as therapies to treat breast cancer. Herceptin is an example.

Necrosis: dead tissue.

Neoadjuvant therapy: treatment with chemotherapy before surgery.

Neupogen: a naturally occurring body chemical that stimulates bone marrow to make more white blood cells, specifically granulocytes or neutrophils, which help defend the body against bacterial and fungal infection.

P53 gene: an important tumor suppressor gene.

Paclitaxel: a chemotherapy drug.

Paget's disease: a type of early breast cancer that involves the nipple.

Palliate: a treatment that is used to control side effects, such as in reducing pain, but not to cure.

Palpable: identifiable by touch. A palpable mass can be identified by touch.

Pamidronate: a drug that can lower high blood calcium levels and that can help strengthen bones and reduce fractures and pain in patients with bone metastases from cancer.

Pathologist: a physician who diagnoses disease through the gross and microscopic evaluation of tissues and cells.

Pathology: the study of disease through gross and microscopic evaluation of tissues and cells.

Pectoralis major: major chest wall muscles.

Pectoralis minor: minor chest wall muscle.

Percent S phase (also S phase fraction): a measurement to discern how rapidly cells are dividing.

Peripheral blood stem cell transplants (PBSCT): a procedure in which young blood cells, called *stem cells,* are collected and reinfused into a patient's bloodstream after high-dose chemotherapy to accelerate the recovery of blood counts.

Phytoestrogens: plant estrogens.

PICC line: IV access for chemotherapy that is inserted into a vein in the forearm.

Ploidy: the number of chromosome sets in a cell with normal cells having the normal 46, or diploid, set of chromosomes and tumor cells often having an abnormal number, or aneuploid, set of chromosomes.

Port-A-Cath: a small device surgically placed under the skin in the upper chest to deliver chemotherapy.

Prolactin: a pituitary hormone that stimulates lactation.

Quadrantectomy: removal of approximately a quarter of the breast in segmental distribution with a simultaneous attempt to clear the margins of a larger breast cancer.

Radiation dosimetrist: a professional who assists the radiation oncologist and who is trained to analyze the contour and shape of the breast in relation to the other organs and prepare a plan on a computer that delineates radiation patterns.

Radiation oncologist: a physician who specializes in using radiation therapy to treat cancer.

Radiation therapy: cancer treatment that uses radiation, a form of energy, to kill cancer cells.

Radio-labeled tracer (gamma-guided radio-labeled tracer): a radioactive tracer used to detect the sentinel node during sentinel node biopsy. The tracer is injected in the breast around the area of the tumor. It travels through the lymphatic channels to the sentinel nodes. The surgeon then uses a handheld gamma detector probe to identify the lymph nodes before making an incision.

Radiologist: a physician trained to diagnose disease using imaging studies, such as mammograms, ultrasound, CT, and MRI.

Raloxifene (Evista): a selective estrogen receptor modulator (SERM) that has been shown to reduce osteoporosis and appears to reduce the chance of developing breast cancer.

Regional recurrence: a recurrence in the skin or chest wall bordering the breast or lymph nodes surrounding the breast area.

Resection: the surgical removal of an area.

Saline implant: a breast implant that contains salt water.

Scleroderma: a collagen vascular disease.

Selective estrogen receptor modulator (SERM): chemical agents that act as an antiestrogen, blocking the estrogen receptor on certain tissues like the breast and that cause an estrogenlike effect on other tissues, such as bone.

Selenium: an antioxidant mineral.

Sentinel node: the first lymph node to which a tumor drains.

Sentinel node mapping: a surgical procedure in which blue dye and/or radio-labeled tracer is injected into the breast tissue around the tumor to locate the lymph node most likely to contain cancer, called the *sentinel node*. This is done to determine if the cancer has spread to the lymph nodes, information that is critical to the staging and treatment of breast cancer.

Serial sectioning: a method of evaluating lymph nodes for tumor deposits.

Silicone implant: a breast implant made using silicone gel.

Staging: a system to classify cancer using the TNM system and resulting in stages defined from Stage I to Stage IV.

Stereotactic core needle biopsy: a type of core needle biopsy that uses computerized mammographic imaging in three dimensions to biopsy a nonpalpable mass or calcification.

Subcuticular: beneath the epidermis.

Supraclavicular lymph nodes: lymph nodes located above the clavicle.

Surgical oncologist: a fellowship-trained surgical specialist, also usually board-certified in general surgery, who deals with the surgical treatment of cancer and its relationship to other treatment modalities.

Systemic recurrence: recurrence of cancer in the distant organs.

Systemic treatment or control: treatment of the whole body to control the spread of cancer. Chemotherapy and hormone therapy are examples.

Tamoxifen: a SERM (selective estrogen receptor modulator) that has been shown to be an effective treatment in hormone-receptor–expressing (estrogen and/or progesterone receptor) breast cancers at all stages of disease. Tamoxifen has also been shown to reduce the development of new breast cancers and to reduce osteoporosis. Tamoxifen causes a slightly increased risk of uterine cancer, apparently unlike Evista.

Telangiectasia: development of small red vessels on the skin, a potential long-term side effect of radiation therapy.

Tissue expander: a deflated implant placed beneath the muscles of the chest wall. It is gradually expanded with fluid to stretch the skin in order to accommodate the final breast implant that will later replace it.

TNM system: a system used to stage cancer: T (tumor size), N (degree of lymph node involvement), and M (degree of metastases, or cancer spread to distant areas of the body).

TRAM flap (transverse abdominal myocutaneous flap): surgery employing skin, fat, and muscle from the lower abdomen to reconstruct the breast after mastectomy.

Triple test: a standard that a breast biopsy must meet to be considered complete and accurate. The findings from the biopsy, the physical examination and the mammogram or ultrasound must all be consistent.

Ultrasound: a noninvasive procedure that uses sound waves to obtain images on a monitor of an area within the body for diagnostic purposes.

Wide excision: see lumpectomy.

Wire localization: also see bracketing wire localization. A procedure in which a radiologist places one or more fine wires into the breast to guide the surgeon in removal of a nonpalpable tumor.

INDEX

Page numbers in *italic* indicate illustrations; those in **bold** indicate tables.